SOCIAL MEDICINE AND MEDICAL SOCIOLOGY IN THE TWENTIETH CENTURY

THE WELLCOME INSTITUTE SERIES IN THE HISTORY OF MEDICINE

Forthcoming Titles

Operative Chymist
Anthony Morson

Ashes to Ashes: The History of Smoking and Health
Stephen Lock (ed.)

Out of Otherness: Characters and Narrators in the Dutch Venereal Disease Debates 1850–1990
Annet Mooij

Academic enquiries regarding the series should be addressed to the editors W. F. Bynum, V. Nutton and Roy Porter at the Wellcome Institute for the History of Medicine, 183 Euston Road, London NW1 2BE, UK

SOCIAL MEDICINE AND MEDICAL SOCIOLOGY IN THE TWENTIETH CENTURY

Edited by Dorothy Porter

Rodopi

Amsterdam – Atlanta, GA 1997

First published in 1997
by Editions Rodopi B. V., Amsterdam – Atlanta, GA 1997.

Design and typesetting by Christine Buckley, the Wellcome Trust.
Printed and bound in The Netherlands by Editions Rodopi B. V.,
Amsterdam – Atlanta, GA 1997.

British Library Cataloguing in Publication Data
A catalogue record for this book is available from the British Library
ISBN 90-420-0346-4 (Paper)
ISBN 90-420-0356-1 (Bound)

Porter, Dorothy
Social Medicine and Medical Sociology
in the Twentieth Century/Dorothy Porter, – Amsterdam – Atlanta,
GA: Rodopi. – ill. (Clio Medica 43 / ISSN 0045-7183;
The Wellcome Institute Series in the History of Medicine)

Front cover:

Still from cartoon "See How They Won", 1935.

In 1935, Boots Pure Drug Company Ltd launched a Winter Health Campaign which focused for the first time on preventative healthcare, encouraging people to buy products such as throat pastilles, children's cough mixture, aspirin and cod liver oil to combat the inevitable winter coughs and colds.

Central to the Campaign was a Hollywood-made cartoon "See How They Won" which was released in cinemas throughout the UK. It was supported by a promotional boardgame, gramophone record, and poster campaign as well as window bills and displays in over 1000 branches of Boots The Chemists.

Details courtesy of *The Boots Company Archive*

Printed in The Netherlands

I dedicate this book to Alexander.

Contents

Introduction

Dorothy Porter

Virgin Territory?

'An exploration of the almost virgin territory which lay between the provinces of the medical and social sciences'[1]

The biometrician and geneticist Francis Crew believed this to be the central aim of the new academic discipline of social medicine founded in Britain in the 1940s. Crew, Professor of Social Medicine at Edinburgh University, had first seen the potential role which the social sciences could play in medicine while he was a Chief M.O. in the services during World War II. Working in the armed forces allowed doctors a unique opportunity to make a study of positive health.[2] 'In the Army,' he argued, 'positive health is no empty phrase; for a purely negative health standard is not good enough for a medical service which is called upon to assess training procedures and to promote and prescribe a regimen appropriate to the maintenance of the highest level of attainable efficiency for an exacting life and an increasing variety of specialised activities imposed by mechanisation.'[3] In the army the term positive health was given an exact meaning. Through various tests of intelligence, agility, endurance, strength, motivation etc. the army aimed to match each recruit to the most appropriate occupational role within the force. Crew explained that this constituted 'a measure of inherent and acquired qualities,' which prevented 'a disharmony between the individual and the conditions of his employment. In the Army as in Civil life much sickness is nothing more or less than disinclination born of dissatisfaction and transformed into disability.'[4] He believed that the marriage of social science and medicine could achieve a similar social biology of health and human ecology for the civilian population too.[5]

Like the first Professor of Social Medicine in Britain, John Ryle, Crew linked medicine as a social science to political reform because both perceived the social sciences to be dedicated to social transformation.[6] Their view was understandable because, from its inception, social science was bound to a prescriptive mission. The earliest attempts to develop a 'social mathematics' and 'social physics' of society were directed at reforming the political operation of power and restructuring of social relations. The reform impulse of early 'social physics' carried over into the first attempts to make medicine a social science in the mid-nineteenth century. Advocates of 'social medicine' at that time invented the physician as an attorney to the poor and encouraged him to take up his duty to participate in the political planning of society. The idea that social science could assist medicine to fulfil a political role in the planning of a future society extended into late-nineteenth-century investigations of social pathology which relied upon eugenics to improve population health. Some late-nineteenth-century public health theorists suggested that medicine should become involved in the corporate planning of communal life by turning itself into 'medicine from the social standpoint.' The idea of social medicine as a form of political and social engineering had a profound legacy for the relations of social science *in* medicine.

Crew's view, therefore, that uniting the medical and the social sciences was crossing 'virgin territory' was rather myopic. Nineteenth-century experiments in social medicine had already achieved that. Furthermore, nineteenth-century sociology was born out of a medical metaphor which compared the analysis of social order to the analysis of living organisms.[7] Sociology, like its social scientific predecessors, was wedded to reordering society but its prescriptive goals were derived from the organic analogy of society. The intellectual objective of the new 'positive' science of the social organism was to identify the laws which governed the harmonious functioning of its organs. Its method was to differentiate normal from pathological social states. The prescriptive nature of the organic analogy continued to have an equally profound influence on the development of the social science *of* medicine.

Let us look for a moment at the political character of the early social sciences and examine the way in which this influenced their relations with medicine. We can begin with the translation of social physics into nineteenth-century political medical programmes. This will provide a background for understanding the mission of social science *in* medicine, or social medicine. An essential background for understanding the development of a social science *of* medicine, or medical sociology, is an analysis of the organic analogy and its differentiation of the normal and the pathological. Perhaps it will then be possible to see, through the work of our essayists here, how these developments remained critical to the relations between medicine and the social sciences in the twentieth century.

Nineteenth-Century Social Medicine and Political Planning

Before the nineteenth century an Enlightenment tradition of applying Newtonian philosophy and Lockean empirical methods to the analysis of society, as a mechanism made up of homogeneous individuals all born equal under the law, attempted to discover the mathematical laws which governed its operations.[8] The *philosophe*, Ambroise Condorcet, believed that politics could become a technocratic exercise rather than an act of will through a system of social mathematics based on a reduction of inequality and diversity.[9] The quantitative analysis of social physics was developed in the early nineteenth century by Lambert-Adolphe-Jaques Quetelet, the Belgian astronomer who devised the theory of the normal frequency distribution curve.[10] A generation younger than Condorcet, Quetelet (1796–1874) dropped the moral science of precepts and made a transition to a social science of laws. But he still believed that social science could provide the basis for reform. While setting up an observatory in Brussels in 1823, Quetelet began to apply the routine methods of mathematical analysis used in astronomical observation to some of the demographic questions which had been investigated by Laplace and Joseph Fourier. This led him to found a social mathematics based upon the concept of the average man being equivalent to the concept of the centre of gravity in celestial physics. He believed that humans were fundamentally alike and that the deviant effects of the peripheral members of the social body cancelled each other out. Virtue was a just mean between two vicious extremes. Quetelet assumed a direct equivalence between the statistical laws of society and the mechanical laws of the heavens and that the historical path of society could be deduced in the same way as that of the planets. His theory of the normal distribution of human variation became a kind of measurement of error, a set of accidental fluctuations from a golden mean.[11] He believed that social statistics could provide the basis of the scientific management of society which chimed with the views of the English political philosopher Jeremy Bentham who believed that scientific government could be achieved through a felicific calculus.[12]

In France in the early nineteenth century the application of social physics did not lead to social reform. Instead it created a new academic inquiry into the conditions which determine health and disease. There had been a long tradition of the use of 'number in medicine' in France. The celebrated philosopher-physician Cabanis had first pointed the way to the possible use of statistics in the investigation of the social origins of disease. The numerical regularities observed by Laplace in astronomy were applied by the alienist Philippe Pinel in the evaluation of therapeutic effectiveness and developed further with regard to physiological inquiries by Pierre Louis. An ex-army surgeon, Louis René Villermé, who was a friend of Quetelet, translated social physics into elaborate studies of the differential mortality of the rich and poor and the health conditions of the proletariat and their average expectation of life. The result was a definitive identification of death as an economic and social disease. The revelation of this relationship, however, did not stimulate political action. Villermé warned against the involvement of the state in health reform and suggested instead that the remoralization of the poor would eliminate epidemic disease and premature mortality.[13]

In France there was no institutionalization of social statistics or health reform in learned societies or political organizations but a distinct group of socio-medical investigators emerged in the early nineteenth century whom William Coleman has called the '*partie d'hygiène*.' Most of them were neither practising physicians nor official bureaucrats nor revolutionary political agitators. They were university-trained 'hygienists' and they completed commissioned studies for a range of agencies from the Ministry of the Interior, to the Royal Medical Academy and the Academy of Moral and Political Sciences. Most hygienists studied under Jean Noel Hallé within the Département d'hygiène of the new Royal Academy of Medicine set up at the end of the Napoleonic Wars. Numerous students became leading lights of the *partie d'hygiène* such as Parent-Duchatelet, Michel Lèvy and Villermé himself.[14]

The reform impulse of social physics was incorporated into the co-option of the social sciences into medicine in the middle years of the nineteenth century. Radical clinicians, like Jules Guérin in revolutionary Paris in 1848 and Rudolf Virchow in Prussia, believed that medicine should adopt a new social scientific profile along with a consciousness of social responsibility and play a political role in the emergent modern state.[15] The idea that social science could assist medicine in developing a social consciousness continued as health increasingly became acknowledged as a social good as well as an individual possession.

Rudolf Virchow and his comrades in the cause of medical reform in Prussia demanded the reduction of unnecessary mortality through complete democracy, universal education and the creation of a new role for the physician as the 'natural attorney to the poor.'[16] When in 1848 the Prussian government employed the future founding father of cellular pathology to investigate an outbreak of typhus fever in the mill district of Upper Silesia, he identified the insanitary conditions in which the weavers lived as the cause of the epidemic. He developed what he chose to call a 'socio-logical' epidemiology which led him to conclude that the strength of the disease amongst the Upper Silesians was due to their subjugated state.[17] Poor and oppressed for decades by the imperial exploitation of Prussia, they had failed to rebel because of widespread ignorance and the socio-psychological apathy which resulted from the culture of poverty and political slavery. The impoverished conditions under which they lived would never have been allowed to develop in a 'free democracy with general self-government.' Therefore, he concluded,[18]

> The logical answer to the question as to how conditions similar to those that have unfolded before our eyes in Upper Silesia can be prevented in the future is, therefore, very easy and simple: education, with its daughters, liberty and prosperity.

So,[19]

> we have thus reached with logical argument the stand-point … [that] … Medicine has imperceptibly led us into the social field and placed us in a position of confronting directly the great problems of our time.

For this reason Virchow had no hesitation in saying that the elimination of famine and ignorance would prevent population decimation from virulent diseases. A well-fed and politically emancipated population would produce a society in which both capital and labour had the same rights to health.[20]

> These are the radical methods I am suggesting as a remedy against the re-occurrance of famine and of great typhus epidemics in Upper Silesia …. May therefore the next interval be used to preserve from the repetition of such scenes of horror by liberal institutions for the benefit of the people, which to the shame of the government has so far been inhabited only by poor and neglected people.

In England attempts at turning medicine into a social science led to social reform from the mid-Victorian period. Doctors were amongst the founders of the National Association for Social Science in 1856 which aimed to create a social science of government. The Association pursued public health reform as a prime target for policy-making based on scientific principles.[21] The quantification of health and disease was critical to making public health policy scientific, with leading reformers using the London Statistical Society as a political platform and establishing the Epidemiological Society for the same purpose. Some members of the English medical profession, such as John Simon and Henry Rumsey, believed that public health policy was the logical place where medicine should play a central role in government. Medical statesmanship would provide citizens with protection from disease as the law provided them with protection against physical violence against their person. English state medicine aimed to provide medical management of social relations and behaviour.[22] By the century's end the Chief Medical Officer of the Local Government Board, Arthur Newsholme, called this 'medicine from the social standpoint,' the purpose of which he perceived as 'the corporate management of communal life.'[23] Newsholme was sufficiently keen on creating medicine from the social standpoint to provide enough education in the social sciences for his students to allow one of them to create the General Registrar's Classification of Occupations which became a principal methodological tool for British sociology.[24]

By the end of the century the conceptualization of medicine as a social science in Germany included beliefs about the biological determination of social behaviour which Newsholme would have rejected because of his opposition to eugenics. Eugenics succeeded bacteriology as the predominant biological rhetoric within discourses on social organization by 1900. The offshoot of this development in Germany was a new movement called social hygiene, the most prominent advocate of which was the physician and reformer, Alfred Grotjahn.[25] Grotjahn incorporated evolutionary theory into an analysis of what he identified as 'social pathology.'[26] From this basis he developed what Paul Weindling has called 'welfare eugenics' aimed at planning a future healthy population by mixing environmental with eugenic reforms.[27] In Germany Darwinian theories of evolution had been embraced, above all, by the monist theorist of ecology, Ernst Haeckel.[28] Although perceived as dated, Haeckel's monism was taken up by the new theorists of racial hygiene in Germany in the early twentieth century.[29] The Racial Hygiene Society was founded in Berlin in 1905[30] and was set up in part as a reaction against the social science orientation of public health and social hygiene developed by reformers such as

Grotjahn.[31] Where social hygiene was influenced by social science, racial hygiene drew upon racial anthropology. However, as Weindling has pointed out, they both shared a common belief in the causal nature of biology in social development and the importance of eugenics to the planned regulation of human reproduction.[32] Their common social-biological approach to health blurred the distinctions between the two movements.[33] Similar developments throughout Europe linked medicine to social planning through the control of human reproduction. In England, where Francis Galton had first created the science of eugenics, voluntary health reform movements multiplied, including the Eugenics Education Society in 1907, which aimed to promote the medical management of the quality of future populations.

Whether in the planning of a eugenically sound society or within the context of the corporate management of communal life, the late nineteenth century identified a new managerial role for medicine and social science in the modern political state. This role continued to be the *raison d'être* of social medicine in the twentieth century.

The Organic, the Normal and the Pathological

The mechanistic model of social physics was not universally accepted by its contemporaries. It was dismissed, for example, by Edmund Burke who used a chemical metaphor to explain the volatile, indeterminate vitality of social and political change.[34] Others believed that society was a functioning organism rather than a physical machine. In *The Order of Things* Michel Foucault suggested that the social sciences succeeded the natural sciences at the turn of the nineteenth century by replacing static analytical taxonomies with functional organic systems.[35] Thus wealth, natural history and grammar transmuted into economics, biology and philology by redefining life, labour and language in terms of the functional discourse of scientific rationality in a modern capitalist society. In what Foucault chose to call the Classical Age of knowledge the subject of objective enquiry was divinely ordained 'nature' but the modern '*episteme*' consisted of the human sciences which focused on the history of man himself.[36] The human sciences reconstructed the functional relations of organic systems hidden beneath classifiable, observable characteristics. Foucault argued, therefore, that objective study of the order of human society translated the language of the natural sciences to the social sciences through an organic metaphor. Organicism was linked to scientism as a defining cultural characteristic of modern society.

The organic metaphor of a functional society powerfully advanced a division between the sociologically normal and the pathological which first emerged in the work of Auguste Comte. Comte's intellectual predecessor in utilizing the organic analogy, Claude-Henri de Saint-Simon,[37] wanted to replace Catholicism and superstition with Newtonian rationalism by applying natural philosophy to the study of social order to discover its natural laws, using the methods of Lockean empiricism. But unlike Condorcet or Quetelet, he did not believe that society was made up of homogeneous, equivalent individuals but was divided into ruling, parasitical and industrial classes,[38] because humanity consisted biologically of thinkers, artists and workers. Society had its own physiology, just like the human body.[39] His concept of social science, therefore, was one which he frequently referred to as social physiology, which Comte later condensed into the term sociology. It is clear from the relationship that Comte's work bears to Saint-Simon that European sociology is grounded in analogical organicist reasoning.[40] But the goal of 'the true Organic Doctrine,' Saint-Simon pointed out, was that it 'can alone produce the harmony so imperatively demanded by the condition of European Society.'[41] The pursuit of a science of society was subsequently linked to the search for political prescriptives and the creation of sociology was part of a programmatic doctrine of positive social unity.[42]

Positive social unity was the central goal of sociology as it was defined by Auguste Comte.[43] Like Saint-Simon, Comte rejected all social philosophies of negation which led to social instability and revolution, such as Hegelianism, and sought to identify the mechanisms of social integration and harmony. He viewed society as an organism governed by laws that resulted in the harmonious functioning of its interdependent organs. The task of a positive science of the social organism was to observe the laws governing social stability. The identification of these laws would synthetically produce a new intellectual order that would result in human unity. The task of sociology was to realize the true positive spirit in history, ending war, conflict and diverse antagonisms.[44] Sociology was a prescriptive as much as a descriptive science that would inaugurate a new era in human history. The era of positive philosophy would replace religion as the dominant ideology upon which the social order depended.[45] Sociology was the course through which the system of positive philosophy would become what T. H. Huxley was later aptly to describe as Catholicism with Christianity taken out.[46]

Comte's positivist sociology has inspired critics such as Herbert Marcuse, Irving Zeitlin and Geoffrey Hawthorn to highlight the authoritarian potential of the application of the organic analogy to the social world.[47] Perhaps the most devastating criticism of Comte came from his younger contemporary, John Stuart Mill.[48] Georges Canguilhem has pointed out, however, that the most significant consequence of Comte's use of the bio-physiological model of positivist inquiry into organic systems was the transfer of the idea of *the normal and the pathological* into the discourse on social behaviour. Positivist social inquiry aimed to identify the normal state of social order determined by the general laws of human unity. Comte used a physiological model of pathological inflammation as a deviation from 'the normal state' of an organ to construct the idea of the sociologically normal. When the doctor, phrenologist and medical theorist, François Joseph Victor Broussais, challenged the ontological notion of illness with a sliding scale between the normal and the pathological, he provided Auguste Comte with the conceptual apparatus for developing a science of the norms and standards of behaviour that made up the basis of society. The fundamental proposition of positivist sociology is that all behaviour is caused and the laws which determine it can be empirically identified and experimentally predicted. Normal social behaviour is that which has followed its determined path. Pathological social behaviour is that which deviates, that is, a variation of the 'normal state.'[49] But as the historian Ian Hacking points out, the term normal can, in the empirical sense, mean typical – quantified, statistically significant, average, median etc. – but also implies a prescriptive value.[50]

In his essay *On the Normal and the Pathological* in 1943 Foucault's teacher, Georges Canguilhem, discussed how the origin of the word normal has both a Latin and a Greek root. The Latin root *norma* means T square which is geometrically orthogonal. The relation of the word normal to the Greek suffix *ortho* is revealing. The normal is often closely related to the orthodox – the 'correct' doctrine or straight version of something. Normal is a value of the orthodox rule as much as it represents a theory of the quantitatively typical.[51] The analysis of normative belief has brought the whole relationship of facts and value into question within sociology but in Comte this relationship was most starkly demonstrated. The 'normal state' of social order, that which creates social unity, became not simply an analysis of what existed, but that which should be sought for through the institution of a positivist ideal. Positivism was, especially in Comte's latter years, a science of social pathology striving to obtain a state of purified social normalcy.[52]

> The positive spirit is the only possible basis for a resolution of the intellectual and moral anarchy that above all characterises the great crisis of our time .... The positive school was gradually prepared, during the revolutionary struggle of the past three centuries, to constitute as much as is possible the true normal state of all the classes and elements of knowledge and of society.

As Hacking points out, Comte illustrates the inherent tension in the concept of the normal as a representation of an existing average and the normal as a figure of perfection to which it is possible to progress.

The organic metaphor of normal and pathological states was extended by Emile Durkheim into an analysis of the causes of normativity itself as the basis of social cohesion, integration and stability. In this context Durkheim explored the normative construction of individuation. He suggested that in modern society, characterized by increasing division of labour, social unity depended upon the successful social construction of individualism. When the socialization of the individual broke down, patterns of social pathology resulted, such as suicide. Suicide, Durkheim argued, was not just an expression of individual despair but a symptom of social disintegration.

Differentiation between the normal and the pathological remained central to the subsequent sociological analysis of social integration forming the conceptual basis, for example, of the sociology of deviance. In socio-medical enquiry, however, the social-biological determination of normal and pathological states has been problematic. The conceptual tensions inherent within the organic metaphor continued to loom large in the development of medical sociology as a discipline, derived, as it was, from the analysis of social integration and deviance.[53]

'Medical Power and Social Knowledge' in the Twentieth Century

Nineteenth-century concepts linking social science, and 'medicine-as-a-social-science,' to social planning provide essential background to understanding the relations between the disciplines in the twentieth century. Our essayists below who examine the emergence of 'social medicine' as an academic discipline show how it co-opted social science into building a healthy and equitable society. The authors here who analyse the development of 'medical sociology,' on the other hand, illustrate how it grew out of the sociological investigations of deviance which were grounded in organicist notions of normal and pathological states. Collectively the chapters demonstrate how promoters of social science *in* and *of* medicine linked their intellectual goals to political missions, most of which were considered by their supporters to be radical and anti-establishment.[54] The essays highlight, however, how radical intentions could produce conservative results.

The essays deal largely with the relationship between medicine and social science in Britain in the twentieth century, but we begin with a discussion of one of the earliest attempts to formally institutionalize it in an interdisciplinary programme of education at the Yale Institute of Human Relations in the 1920s. Teaching in social medicine began as early as 1902 with some lectures being given by Martin Kirchner, a Professor of Hygiene at the Berlin medical school. It was further developed by Grotjahn when he was given an independent chair of social medicine at Berlin by the socialist government after the First World War, but it was discontinued by the conservative medical faculty after his death in 1931.[55] A comprehensive experiment was tried in the 1920s at Yale when the 'Institute of Human Relations' was set up by James Rowland Angell, President of the University, and Milton C. Winternitz, Dean of the medical school, aimed at creating new pathways for interdisciplinary education and research. In the article on 'Milton C. Winternitz and the Yale Institute of Human Relations: A Brief Chapter in the History of Social Medicine,' reproduced here from *The Yale Journal of Biology and Medicine*,[56] the late Arthur Viseltear identified the roots of the Yale experiment in the institutionalization of the social sciences, not only in the universities, but also in the National Research Council in the USA set up after the First World War. The programmes of interdisciplinary studies supported by the National Research Council included medicine as a social science.[57] At the turn of the century the University of Chicago perpetuated the Enlightenment belief in the social sciences as vehicles for promoting social, economic and political reform. A new philosophy of the academy grew up at Chicago which advocated that it should assist a better understanding of society and help resolve problems such as waste, inefficiency and societal and personal maladjustment. Angell and Winternitz both came from Chicago University and believed that the social sciences would force the University to extend its resources and consider community and societal problems of a practical nature. The Chicago school philosophy echoed some of the hopes of Comtian positivism when it suggested that it was the responsibility of the University to break down barriers between departments, programmes and schools and provide the human engineering necessary for the organization of social harmony. When Angell became president in 1921 he wanted Yale to serve the needs of society rather than be an academic ivory tower. Winternitz's agenda fitted in with Angell's goals because he believed medicine was a social science and that medical students should become concerned not just with diseased organs but with the whole man, not only with sickness but with health, not only with biology but with the entire social and economic environment.[58] Winternitz complained that technological advances in medicine had divided up the physical organism of the patient, creating unnecessary proliferation of medical specialities. Medicine had been diverted from the patient to his pathology – the old-fashioned doctor was a generalist who knew all about his patient's passion for fishing, his son Billy etc. The old family physician knew his patients in a different way, holistically. Individuals were not just aggregations of cells but whole persons who lived in a society, worked, married, had children, were happy or unhappy, and encountered disease. This philosophical critique of technological, specialist medicine was shared by contemporary US reformers within medical education and public health such as Richard Cabot and Charles Winslow, who also focused on the individual and his social environment.[59] Viseltear discusses, however, how, despite enthusiasm plus $7million of funding from the Russell Sage Foundation, the experiment at the Yale Institute of Human Relations failed through lack of co-operation amongst the faculty and the desire amongst students to opt for an education in high-tech rather than social medicine.

Winternitz's critique of technological, specialist medicine was mirrored in the social medicine movement in Europe, especially in the UK,[60] but turning medicine into a social science became bound up with the politics of the state in the 1940s in Britain. The creation of social medicine as an academic discipline reaffirmed nineteenth-century beliefs about the political responsibilities of medicine when it became a central issue of educational reform in Britain from the late 1930s. Nigel Oswald, in 'Training Doctors for the National Health Service: Social Medicine, Medical Education and the GMC 1936–48,' argues that the enthusiasm for educational reform amongst a powerful group of elite medical academics and civil servants within the Ministry of Health at this time was directly linked to the planning of the National Health Service, which began in earnest from 1936.[61] An odd group of bed fellows which included the highly conservative Regius Professor of Medicine at Oxford, Sir Edward Farquhar Buzzard, and the equally radical Regius Professor of Physic at Cambridge, John Alfred Ryle, plus Lord Nuffield of Morris Motors and the leading medical civil servant of the day, Sir Wilson Jameson, conspired to influence the medical curriculum in order to produce a new type of general practitioner to run the new service. The GP was to take on a new role in nationalized medicine as a health promoter. Social medicine would produce general practitioners who were interested as much in the causes of ill-health and their prevention as in the therapeutic treatment of disease. Such a preventive general practitioner would use the nationalization of medical services as an opportunity to institute a new campaign to improve the health of the population, taking over where the Medical Officer of Health left off. The role of the MOH by this time concentrated largely on the management of services and environmental health control.[62] Ryle, who became the first Professor of Social Medicine at the new Institute set up at Oxford with Nuffield funding, also saw social medicine as a route to rehumanizing the discipline, counteracting the increasing technologization of specialist therapeutic practice.[63]

Oswald suggests that the consensus which surrounded the planning of the health service and the reform of medical education that had built up during the war disintegrated after 1945 as sectional interests fought bitter battles over status, salaries and political control within the new system. As a result the debate about medical education was pushed to the periphery along with social medicine's goal of reconstructing the general practitioner. But beyond medicine itself, academics from associated fields who were involved in the analysis of health and social policy were also attempting to define the new discipline.[64]

In 'Making Medicine Social: The Case of the Two Dogs with Bent Legs,' Ann Oakley outlines the political nature of the broader intellectual context which contributed to the development of social medicine in Britain. She points out that, as J. B. S. Haldane illustrated in *Heredity and Politics* in 1938,[65] there was a general enthusiasm amongst some British intellectuals at that time for applying new knowledge of human biology to social organization, but a major obstacle remained the question of the relative influence of nature and nurture. For example, genetics could show differences rather than resemblances and could tell you why one mouse was black and the other white but could not tell you why both were mice. Being unable to provide determining causal explanations, human genetics could not differentiate between the relative roles played by heredity or malnutrition, nature or nurture, in creating two dogs with bent legs. In human populations the dilemma was compounded where both natural and social/environmental causes for biological variation were especially difficult to discern. Oakley claims that this was a crucial theme in social medicine in the late 1930s and early 1940s as it challenged biological-determinist views of health. Countering biological-determinist claims provided a powerful impetus in two ways: theories underlying medicine and health and disease were forced to take the social into account; and a new awareness of the social relations of health and disease emphasized the need to socialize medical practice, i.e., justify the creation of non-profit- making service provision accessible to all – a state-funded health service.

In this context Oakley discusses her father's (Richard Titmuss) contribution to social medicine in which social class as a determinant of health was a persistent issue. Titmuss was a self-educated actuary who eventually became Professor of Social Administration at the London School of Economics as the result of his statistical analysis of social welfare and its relationship to the development of social policy. Oakley argues that in the first half of the century public discourses on health were heavily influenced by eugenics, focusing on the quality of population as a major public health concern.[66] The Eugenics Society embraced people from widely divergent social backgrounds and an allegiance to eugenics had become equated with a commitment to social reform.[67] By the late 1930s British eugenists tried, for obvious reasons, to distance themselves from German policy and it was at this point that Titmuss became involved.[68] In 1937, working as an inspector for a large insurance company in London, he was also developing a career as a statistician. He joined the Eugenics Society in 1937 and subsequently became a member of Council and editor of the *Eugenics Review*. In publications such as *Poverty and Population* he attempted to demonstrate the level of premature mortality resulting from environmental and preventable causes; and from 1938, acting on behalf of the Population Investigation Committee of the Eugenics Society, he tried to persuade the Registrar-General, Sir Sylvanus Vivian, to improve official statistics. He was also recruited by Maurice Newfield, editor of the *Eugenics Review*, to try and help fulfil the request of Lord Horder, the President of the Society in 1939, to create a new public image of eugenics. This distanced itself from Nazi Germany and emphasized butter not guns; genes not blood, and the health of the individual rather than the rights of the state. Titmuss discussed with Newfield how the major difficulty involved was dealing with reactionaries whom he described as medieval-minded bigots who used eugenics to justify hostility toward the lower orders of society and the development of social services from which these could benefit. Titmuss's work for the Eugenics Society was, Oakley suggests, epidemiological and sociographic rather than sociological, concerned with the social conditions which produced health outcomes. And it was here that Titmuss rooted the idea of social medicine in the instrument of the social survey as a means of collecting information from and about individuals relevant to health, which was needed to supplement crude mortality data in order to give a wider picture of health. Teaming up with Jerry Morris in 1941, he joined a group called the Committee for the Study of Social Medicine which met under the chairmanship of Professor A. St G. Huggett at St Mary's Hospital. Titmuss started to use the term social medicine in 1942 and within his own research it was part of an ambitious project, conceived with Morris, in which statistical and other forms of social research could reshape both health policy and medical practice. The goal of the new discipline was to have a health-promoting impact on the welfare of the community at large. John Ryle acknowledged their work as the first example of practical social medicine.[69]

Oakley suggests that in the context of her father's work social medicine arose out of a crisis in eugenic thought about health, the move towards state-funded health service and the 'visionary circumstances of world-wide war.' But, she argues, social medicine's commitment to influencing policy-making made it vulnerable to changing political climates and was responsible for its demise.

By contrast Dorothy Porter, in 'The Decline of Social Medicine in Britain in the 1960s,' suggests that the institutional status of social medicine declined in Britain because it lost its original political character. She examines the institutional life of the discipline within the post-war world of academic infighting within medicine and public health. Here we find an embattled discipline, struggling within the university and the medical school to establish both its relevance to the education of doctors on the one hand, and its independent intellectual status from medicine on the other. The Society for Social Medicine was set up in the 1950s by academics who tried to create a scholarly forum for teachers and researchers in the field. The Society's membership was restricted but included both medically trained and non-medically trained academics. Porter argues that social medicine in the 1950s and 1960s ignored the post-war theoretical disputes of the social sciences and uncritically embraced a quantitative paradigm. Furthermore, she suggests that addressing policy-making became a goal secondary to the priority of achieving academic respect. Both of these developments meant that practitioners of the discipline were ill-equipped to negotiate from a position of strength when the re-organization of the health service created a new Faculty of Community Medicine in 1972. Community medicine invented a new paradigm of prevention which emphasized the blending of theory with the practical concerns of service management and left social medicine intellectually isolated and institutionally weak.[70]

If social medicine was institutionally undermined by the creation of community medicine then its prerogative for defining the intellectual relationship between medicine and the social sciences was also under threat by the end of the 1950s with the emergence of another academic discipline, medical sociology. In 'Social Medicine and Medical Sociology 1950–1970: The Testimony of a Partisan Participant,' Margot Jefferys provides a unique insight into the experience of sociologists entering the medical field in the post-war period.[71] Her own entrance into the world of social medicine was via public health teaching, which began to open up to social science in the 1950s assisted by individuals such as John Brotherston, Professor of Public Health first at the London School of Hygiene and Tropical Medicine and later at Edinburgh University. At LSHTM he set up the Oxehy project, funded with Rockefeller money to investigate the effects on health of living on a large council housing estate. As divisions of social medicine spread in other university departments and medical schools they began to reflect the new approach to the role of medicine in prevention which had been stimulated by the work of Ryle and Titmuss and others, with major advances being achieved in the statistical field, especially by the work of Austin Bradford Hill.

Social science in Britain in the 1950s was itself poorly supported. Neither Oxford nor Cambridge University had a sociology department. By contrast anthropology had established a powerful influence in the British university system within the context of an imperialist culture, and retained a deep hostility to the academic institutionalization of any rival social sciences.[72] A few institutions had established departments of sociology before and after World War II, such as that of the London School of Economics, still chaired by Morris Ginsberg with his philosophical approach.[73] A more empirically-based analysis of social structure was beginning to gain ground at the LSE as a result of the appointment of David Glass to a chair.[74] Little interest, however, was shown by any mainstream sociologists in health status or health-related behaviour as social variables or in health services as social institutions. But proponents of social medicine and of a new vision of the public health mission did find a more favourable response from a peculiarly British brand of social investigators who called themselves 'social scientists.' These were an eclectic group trained in economics, economic history or political science who moved into academic departments which encouraged them to study issues associated with poverty and the means of alleviating it. Jefferys acknowledges the important influence of Richard Titmuss in this regard. Notwithstanding a variety of intellectual approaches amongst them, this group was nevertheless bound to the study of health usually through an interest in Marxism, or Fabian Socialism, and wanted to make a contribution to the planned allocation of health resources. A quantitative empirical method of analysis was also a prominent feature amongst them.[75]

Despite various research initiatives and the creation of the Society for Social Medicine, professional opportunities were bleak for social scientists working within a medical or public health education context and most went back to mainstream social science by the early 1960s. Jefferys suggests that the 1964 Todd Commission reaffirmed the idea that social science had no role in the training of doctors when it recommended that any contribution from sociology to medical education should be made by behavioural scientists employed in university departments. The Commission suggested that if social scientists were employed within medical schools they would lose their intellectual identity with their parent discipline. Jefferys herself disagreed with this view, believing that if the subject was to gain legitimation then those who taught it should be immersed in the medical enterprise. Since that time, however, the employment of social scientists within medical schools has spread throughout the British system and the General Medical Council has produced new guidelines about the necessity of introducing the subject into the curriculum. British medical schools now employ their own social scientists rather than liaising with university departments, and some of these appointments currently carry the prestige of readerships and chairs.

Jefferys highlights the institutional dilemmas of medical sociology. Alternatively Uta Gerhardt draws out the intellectual contradictions created by 'The Dilemma of Social Pathology.' She outlines how medical sociology grew out of an organicist analysis of deviance as a type of social pathology which aimed to identify the means of re-integrating the deviant into an harmonious relationship with society. Within the social sciences Gerhardt locates the origin of the concept of social pathology in the early work of the Chicago school of sociology where it was used to describe the idea of individual and social maladjustment.[76] So for example when Stuart Queen and Delbert Mann published *Social Pathology* in 1925,[77] they analysed the social causes and consequences of addiction, deafness, alcoholism, suicide, divorce, illegitimacy, homelessness, old age and mental breakdown, which they perceived as areas of non-integration which required corrective measures. They tried to account for the social disintegration caused by poverty, parental neglect or other unfavourable social conditions during socialization which could make it practically impossible for an adolescent to fit into society. In a characteristically Progressivist sociological analysis, Queen and Mann asserted that social reform had to be a community effort targeted at counteracting social pathology. Social work and education were needed to supplement individual effort and then society could be made an adequate life-world to live in. These ideas remained central to social pathological research and when Queen published the revised edition in World War II with Jennette Gruener,[78] it was re-titled *Obstacles to Social Participation.*

In addition to the idea of individual social maladjustment, John Gillin in *Social Pathology* in 1933[79] identified causes which could lead to a pathological society, such as the natural lack of ability in individuals to keep pace with changing ideals and institutions of society or the failure of society to keep pace in its functional machinery. As a result whole societies could become pathological, but more often just one particular class of people within a social group, or a defective function of government, could cause pathological maladjustment.

Gerhardt suggests that the assumptions of this Progressivist sociology were questioned by a new relativism in the 1940s. Authors such as Richard Fuller[80] began to emphasize the normative basis of deviancy in which moral problems were defined by social values so that, for example, race prejudice was acceptable in some societies and viewed as pathological in others. For Fuller the difference between the normal and the pathological was defined only by social values. This new relativism attempted to replace the moralistic nature of earlier studies of social pathology with a sound scientific approach. Fuller was supported by authors such as Guy Brown who in 1942[81] argued that the solution to social pathology could be found in social scientific research which used the same procedures for analysing both normal and abnormal activities with neutral objectivity. Into this discussion social analysts such as Edwin Lemert[82] introduced the theories of symbolic interactionism[83] which asserted that sociopathic behaviour was created through the identification by others of abnormality. Sociopathic individuation was the reaction of the deviant to societal reaction to them. Sociopathic behaviour was not an intention but a consequence of this set of interactions. Lemert concluded that labelling people deviant alienated them further from society.

The model of deviance as labelling[84] began to dominate post-war studies such as Howard Becker's *Outsiders* and Erving Goffman's[85] work which argued that deviant behaviour was a label rather than a motivation, a stigma aimed at exclusion. Sociologists subsequently took up the side of the deviant. The deviant was presented by sociologists in the 1960s as a powerless underdog confronted by all-powerful societies. Labelling theory was incorporated into the study of the social relations of medicine within the context of the examination of doctors as part of the sociology of the professions. In this context Eliot Freidson's analysis of medical power and Talcott Parsons' theory of the sick-role were seminal.[86] This essentially normative model of medicine both as a theory and as a set of social relations was taken up by sociologists such as Margaret Stacey in the 1970s to develop an interactionist sociology of health-illness conceptions and behaviour.[87]

Interactionism, however, could not provide an explanation of the ontological status of illness. Thus Gerhardt wants to suggest that medical sociology was stuck with the dilemma of social pathology whose theoretical assumptions created an ontological paradox. As a humanist discipline medical sociology, based upon the concept of social pathology, proclaims the relativity of illness labels. Scientific agencies – such as medicine – only curtail the freedom and authenticity of the individual. But the dilemma is that at the same time as the society–individual dichotomy is endorsed, the claim is made that the empirical reality of medical life-worlds can be observed in an objective way. The relativism of interactionism, or constructionism,[88] failed, however, to allow medical sociology to distinguish between pathological and non-pathological social systems or systems of social regulation. Talcott Parsons had distinguished two forms of social control: one resulted in the integration of society through voluntary conformity of members with the community who democratically accepted norms through insight and commitment; the second type of social control was repressive wherein society's functioning was achieved by forcing individuals to comply with rules that could call for rather than discourage deviance. Medicine, for Parsons therefore, was an example of democratic social control.

Gerhardt suggests that the only way to move beyond the dilemma of social pathology is to establish a sociology which distinguishes between pathological and democratic social systems. Sociology must recognize that while some social systems may possess some pathological tendencies they are primarily democratic and distinguishable from pathological authoritarian states such as

Fascism. Such a distinction would prevent sociology from disregarding the question of balance between freedom and necessity and would also lead to an understanding of illness as a reality and not just a medical label.

Gerhardt illustrates the limitations which prescriptive organicist and relativist reasoning has forced upon medical sociology. In 'The Social Space of Illness' David Armstrong argues, by contrast, that medical sociology has expanded its power to discipline the social relations of health and illness and has extended the medical gaze.[89] Historians of medicine have claimed that economic imperatives have produced specialist division of labour within it as a theoretical and practical system,[90] whereas medics themselves claim that specialization resulted from the natural growth of knowledge. But Armstrong argues that the conceptual division of the body into separate localities was the prerequisite for specialization which produced clinical practice organized around localized pathological lesions. The conceptual model of illness underpinning the system of clinical practice which first emerged at the end of the eighteenth century identified pathological lesions on the basis of the clinical examination. These techniques analysed the three-dimensional volume of the body wherein the disease was hidden, and specialization was addressed to the subdivisions of the space or volume of the body.

Armstrong points out that this model of specialization cannot account, however, for the emergence of social medicine as a speciality because social medicine is not related to the analysis of corporal space. Public health practice, with its focus on the environment which surrounded the body, delineated even more clearly the margin and limits of the three-dimensional volume of the body by deploying a web of surveillance around the well-defined contours of the living body. But a new perspective on the nature of illness which emerged in the twentieth century suggested that the threat to health was not the space surrounding the body but other bodies. Bacteriology, which identified interpersonal hygiene as the source of disease, together with new theories of the neurosis underlying mental illness, stressed that illness was the product of past and present relationships.[91] Physiological and psychological medicine now dealt with the interstices of the social, the space between bodies. Social medicine dealt with the space in which the interrelationship between bodies took place, the interactions of bodies, and tracked an unfolding of psycho-social space. This psycho-social space created other disciplines like psychology and sociology, and alliances emerged such as that between psychology and medicine, producing psychological medicine.

Beyond this, medical sociology achieved further disciplinary consolidation within the social space of illness. Illness was no longer a corporeal lesion but a characteristic of a community which required the social survey to map.[92] According to Armstrong, medical sociology transformed the patient. In pathological medicine the patient was no more than the repository of the lesion but in the twentieth century social medicine acknowledged the patient as an actor by recognizing the importance of regimes of personal hygiene and by focusing concern upon patient defaulters from treatment, particularly venereal disease therapies. Health education encouraged active participation of the people themselves in the control of disease and they became the agents of health practice. Non-participation became a central study, such as the low take-up of polio vaccine, or lack of community response to X-ray services for tuberculosis. At the beginning of the twentieth century human behaviour was popularly believed to be determined by biological instinct but, Armstrong asserts, by the 1950s sociology argued successfully that it was governed by belief. Medical sociology produced a new model of the intentionally active patient reflected in concepts such as Talcott Parsons' theory of the 'sick-role.'[93] At one time transition to patient status occurred when they came under the care of the doctor, but sociology now blurred definitions of the boundaries between patienthood and personhood. Potential patienthood was extended to everyone as social science recruited all social actors into the medical enterprise. This was clearly expressed in post-World War II socio-medical surveys where rigid distinctions between health and illness became meaningless since they identified everyone as being at risk from something or other. In 1960 Mechanic and Volkart[94] weakened the distinction between patient and person even further by introducing the concept of illness behaviour which extended to all areas of experience. Armstrong concludes that social medicine and medical sociology crystallized a new illness-space, beyond socio-physical spaces between bodies, where the abstracted products of social activities feed back and jeopardize health, such as the damage done to the ozone layer, radiation, nuclear facilities etc. The relationship between the medical and the social sciences, therefore, Armstrong suggests, has enhanced the web of surveillance achieved by the medical gaze by synthesizing the social and the subjective.

Armstrong uses a Foucaultian analysis[95] to argue that medical sociology has been integral to the expansion of medicine's disciplinary power of surveillance. As discussed earlier, Foucault suggested that, at the turn of the nineteenth century, the social sciences expanded the power of scientific rationality to create a disciplinary society based on new modes of ideological surveillance. Armstrong agrees and suggests that medical sociology has intensified what Herbert Marcuse referred to as 'the logic of domination.' Bryan Turner believes, alternatively, that Foucault's influence upon medical sociology has facilitated the analysis of the moral regulation of medicine itself. In 'Medicine, Diet and Moral Regulation: Foucault's Impact on Medical Sociology,' Turner argues that while medical sociology has achieved a degree of academic success, it lacks theoretical coherence and as a result has made little contribution to the analytical and conceptual development of general sociology. Despite the origins of sociology in medical reasoning in the nineteenth century none of the classical founders of the discipline, except Durkheim, concentrated on illness but focused instead on the social analysis of work, religion and the growth of bureaucratic organizations.[96] Initially sociology in medicine largely accepted the medical model of disease and only when medical sociologists began to develop a sociology of health and illness did the discipline become less committed to the goals of the medical profession and instead integrate its analyses into the broader discipline of sociology through a greater concern with the philosophical underpinnings of disease and illness.[97] Within this context Talcott Parsons' theory of the sick-role was a significant departure since he used it as a means for redefining the analytical paradigm of deviance and social control. As a result, medical sociology subsequently challenged the medical model of disease and tried to develop an effective alternative explanatory system for understanding sickness.[98] Thus medical sociologists frequently became committed to social medicine as an alternative to individualistic allopathic practice and became interested in alternative healing as a critique of the mainstream assumptions of Western medicine.

Like Gerhardt and Armstrong, Turner highlights the importance of Parsons' role in the creation of an independent theoretical basis to medical sociology but this was overtaken by the impact of Foucault's analysis of power in creating a sociology of the body.[99] Parsons and Foucault provided descriptions of institutions of normative coercion such as the law, religion and medicine which exercised discipline over individual behaviour through the exercise of surveillance over everyday life. Actions were both produced and constrained by them and thus such belief systems achieved a hegemonic coercive authority which was often disguised and masked by their normative involvement. In this sense both Parsons and Foucault shared a continuity with Weber's study of rationalization as an historical process.[100]

But Turner admits that sociology is itself another intellectual discipline of industrial society which sought to provide that society with a means of understanding itself. Despite its radical pretensions it is just as much a form of disciplinary knowledge as any other produced by capitalist society, and in one sense is merely another form of rationalization. Because sociology is a product of modernism, Turner suggests that in the post-modern world it has little function where history as a sequence of events has come to an end.

At the heart of the discussions presented in this volume, therefore, is an analysis of the relationship between social-scientific knowledge both *in* and *of* medicine[101] and the sources of social power.[102] They are cautionary tales about naive idealism which hoped that interdisciplinary creativity would lead to either educational or broader political reform. Interdisciplinary conflict rather than creativity often served instead to reinforce the status quo. The essays have also interrogated the critical assault which social science has made upon the dominance of the biomedical model of disease, sickness and health. They have discussed the consequences of what Raymond Illsley suggested occurred when sociology emancipated itself from the status of an under- labourer and achieved 'observer status.'[103] A number of the essayists agree that Parsons' theory of the sick-role was critical to that process by promoting an analysis of the normative basis of the social relations of doctors and patients, health and illness and the functional role of medical knowledge and the medical profession in modern society. Subsequently the self-proclaimed responsibility of medical sociology has been critically to appraise medicine as social interaction and it has represented itself as a radical underdog nipping at the heels of the vastly privileged establishment of medicine as a system of social organization and mobilization of power. But the organic metaphor of the normal and the pathological contradicted such a radical agenda. The authors here have addressed the consequences of the cultural interaction between medicine and social science in the twentieth century by trying to evaluate its significance for the moral and material role of medicine in modern societies. More than anything else they illustrate that the respective power of biology and culture in determining human behaviour and social transition continues to be an unresolved paradox.

Notes

1. F. A. E. Crew, 'Social Medicine as an Academic Discipline,' in Arthur Massey (ed.), *Modern Trends in Public Health* (London: Butterworth, 1949), 46–79, p. 66.
2. Lancelot Hogben, 'Francis Albert Eley Crew, 1886–1973,' *Biographical Memoirs of the Fellows of the Royal Society*, 20 (1974), 135–53.
3. F. A. E. Crew, 'Social Medicine as an Academic Discipline,' *Lancet*, ii (1944), 618.
4. *Ibid.*., 619.
5. Crew, *op.cit.* (ref. 1), 77.
6. See D. Porter, 'The Decline of Social Medicine,' below.
7. See Ian Hacking, *The Taming of Chance* (Cambridge: Cambridge University Press, 1990); Theodore M. Porter, 'Natural Science and Social Theory,' in R. C. Olby *et al.* (eds), *Companion to the History of Modern Science* (London: Routledge, 1990), 1024–44.
8. *Ibid.*.
9. Henry Vyverberg, *Human Nature, Cultural Diversity and the French Enlightenment* (Oxford: Oxford University Press, 1989), 20–33.
10. Gerd Gigerenzer *et al., The Empire of Chance* (Cambridge: Cambridge University Press, 1989), 38–45.
11. Hacking, *op.cit.* (ref. 7), 105–14.
12. Janet Semple, 'Bentham's Utilitarianism and the Provision of Medical Care,' in Dorothy Porter and Roy Porter (eds), *Doctors, Politics and Society: Historical Essays* (Amsterdam and Atlanta: Rodopi, 1993), 30–46. See also Porter, *op.cit.* (ref. 7) and Hacking, *op.cit.* (ref. 7). For further discussion of the rise of statistics and probability theory see *idem, The Rise of Statistical Thinking, 1820–1900* (Princeton: Princeton University Press, 1986); Lorraine J. Daston, *Classical Probability in the Enlightenment* (Princeton: Princeton University Press, 1988); Gerd Gigerenzer *et al., op.cit.* (ref. 10), 38–45. For development of population analysis and statistics in Britain see Patricia James, *Population Malthus. His Life and Times* (London: Routledge & Kegan Paul, 1979), 40–78; Catherine Gallagher, 'The Body Versus the Social Body in the Works of Thomas Malthus and Henry Mayhew,' in Catherine Gallagher and Thomas Laqueur (eds), *The Making of the Modern Body. Sexuality and Society in the Nineteenth Century* (Berkeley: University of California Press, 1987), 83–106; Donald MacKenzie, *Statistics in Britain, 1865–1930: The Social Construction of Scientific Knowledge* (Edinburgh: Edinburgh University Press, 1981); John Eyler, *Victorian Social Medicine* (Baltimore: Johns Hopkins University Press, 1979), 97–122, 123–59; Karl H. Metz, 'Social Thought and Social Statistics in the Early Nineteenth-Century.

The Case of Sanitary Statistics in England,' *International Review of History*, 29 (1984), 254–73. For social statistics and epidemiology in France see W. Coleman, *Yellow Fever in the North. The Methods of Early Epidemiology* (Madison, Wis: University of Wisconsin Press, 1987), 79–107; *idem, Death is a Social Disease* (Madison: Wisconsin: University of Wisconsin Press, 1982),149–80, 277–306.

13. See Coleman, *Death is a Social Disease, op.cit.* (ref. 12); Erwin Ackerknecht, 'Villermé and Quetelet,' *Bulletin for the History of Medicine,* 26 (1952), 317–29. 'Queteletism' did lead to sanitary reform in other European contexts. See for example the discussion of the Netherlands by Eddy Houwart, 'Medical Statistics and Sanitary Provisions: A New World of Social Relations and Threats to Health,' *Tractrix. Yearbook for the History of Science, Medicine, Technology and Mathematics*, 5 (1993/4), 1–33.
14. See Coleman, *Death is a Social Disease, op.cit.* (ref. 12); Matthew Ramsey, 'Public Health in France,' in D. Porter (ed.), *The History of Public Health and the Modern State* (Amsterdam and Atlanta: Rodopi, 1994), 45–118.
15. D. Porter, 'Public Health,' in W. F. Bynum and Roy Porter (eds), *The Routledge Encyclopaedia of the History of Medicine* (London: Routledge, 1993), 1231–61.
16. George Rosen, 'What is Social Medicine?,' *Bulletin of the History of Medicine*, 21 (1947), 674–733. See also D. Porter and R. Porter, 'What Was Social Medicine? An Historiographical Essay,' *Journal of Historical Sociology*, 1 (1988), 90–106; Paul Weindling, 'Was Social Medicine Revolutionary? Virchow on Famine and Typhus in 1848,' *Bulletin of the Society for the Social History of Medicine*, 34 (1984), 13–18.
17. Rudolf Virchow, *Public Health Reports,* edited by L. J. Rather (Maryland: Science History Publications, 1986), 2 vols, Vol. 1, 307–19.
18. *Ibid..*, 318.
19. *Ibid..*
20. *Ibid..*
21. L. Goldman, 'A Peculiarity of the English? The Social Science Association and the Absence of Sociology in Nineteenth-Century Britain,' *Past and Present*, 114 (1987), 133–71.
22. Dorothy Porter, 'Public Health and Centralisation: The Victorian State,' in Roger Detels *et al.* (eds), *Third Oxford Text Book of Public Health,* 2 vols. (Oxford: Oxford University Press, 1997), Vol.1, 19–54.
23. Newsholme quoted by D. Porter, '"Enemies of the Race": Biologism, Environmentalism and the Public Health in Edwardian England,' *Victorian Studies*, 34 (2) (1991), 159–78.

24. Simon Szreter, *Fertility, Class and Gender in Britain 1860–1940* (Cambridge: Cambridge University Press, 1996), 238–82.
25. Paul Weindling, 'Public Health,' in Dorothy Porter (ed.), *The History of Public Health and the Modern State* (Amsterdam and Atlanta: Rodopi, 1994), 119–31. Weindling points out, however, that there were almost as many theories of social hygiene in Germany as theoreticians. For a condensed history of social hygiene in Europe see René Sand, *The Advance to Social Medicine* (London: Staples Press, 1952), 185–294; see also Rosen, *op.cit.* (ref. 16).
26. Alfred Grotjahn, S*ociale Pathologie. Versuch einer Lehre von den sozialen Beziehungen der menschlichen Krankheiten als Grundlage der sozialen Medizin und der sozialen Hygiene* (Berlin: August Hirschwald Verlag, 1915).
27. Paul Weindling, *Health, Race and German Politics Between National Unification and Nazism 1870–1945* (Cambridge: Cambridge University Press, 1989), 370–3, 378–9.
28. Robert J. Richards, *Darwin and the Emergence of Evolutionary Theories of Mind and Behaviour* (Chicago: Chicago University Press, 1978); *idem, The Meaning of Evolution: The Morphological Construction and Ideological Reconstruction of Darwin's Theory* (Chicago: Chicago University Press, 1992).
29. D. Gasman, *The Scientific Origins of National Socialism: Social Darwinism in Ernst Haeckel and the German Monist League* (London: Macdonald, 1971).
30. Weindling, *op.cit.* (ref. 27), 141–2.
31. *Ibid.*, 139; see also Sand, *op.cit.* (ref. 25), 517–20.
32. Weindling, *op.cit.* (ref. 27), 223–6, 370–83.
33. *Ibid.*., 223.
34. Issac Kramnick, *The Rage of Edmund Burke* (New York: Basic Books, 1977); Stephen K. White, *Edmund Burke: Modernity, Politics, and Aesthetics* (Calif., Thousand Oaks: Sage Publications,1994); Peter J. Stanlis, *Edmund Burke: The Enlightenment and Revolution* (New Brunswick, N.J.: Transaction Books, 1991); Stanley Ayling, *Edmund Burke: His Life and Opinions* (London: Cassell 1990); Daniel E. Ritchie (ed.), *Edmund Burke: Appraisals and Applications* (Brunswick, N.J.: Transaction Books, 1990).
35. Michel Foucault, *The Order of Things. An Archeology of the Human Sciences* (London: Tavistock, 1970); *idem, An Archeology of Knowledge*, translated by A. M. Sheridan Smith (London: Tavistock, 1972).
36. *Ibid.*.
37. Geoffrey Hawthorn, *Enlightenment and Despair. A History of Sociology* (Cambridge: Cambridge University Press, 1976), 66–89; Raymond

Aron, *Main Currents in Sociological Thought* (Harmondsworth: Penguin, 1965), 63–109; Irving M. Zeitlin, *Ideology and the Development of Sociological Theory* (Englewood Cliffs, New Jersey: Prentice-Hall, 1968), 56–79; Keith Michael Baker, *Condorcet. From Natural Philosophy to Social Mathematics* (Chicago: University of Chicago Press, 1982), 129–94; H. Stuart Hughes, *Consciousness and Society. The Reorientation of European Social Thought 1890–1930* (Brighton, Sussex: Harvester, 1979), 33–66.

38. Ghita Ionescu (ed.), *Saint-Simon, Claude-Henri de Rouvroy. The Political Thought of Saint-Simon* (Oxford: Oxford University Press, 1976).
39. Frank E. Manuel, *The New World of Henri Saint-Simon* (Cambridge, Mass.: Harvard University Press, 1956).
40. See Theodore Porter, *op.cit.* (ref. 7), 1030–4.
41. Hawthorn, *op.cit.* (ref. 37).
42. *Ibid.*, 66–89.
43. Auguste Comte, *Cours de philosophie positive* (Paris: Bachelier, 1830–1842).
44. Mary Pickering, *Auguste Comte: An Intellectual Biography* (Cambridge: Cambridge University Press, 1993).
45. Keneth Thompson (ed.), *Auguste Comte: The Foundation of Sociology* (London: Nelson 1976).
46. Theodore Porter, *op.cit.* (ref. 7), 1033.
47. Hacking, *op.cit.* (ref. 7), 160–9; Hawthorn, *op.cit.* (ref. 37); Herbert Marcuse, *Reason and Revolution* (London: Routledge, 1986 [1941]), 340–60.
48. J. S. Mill, *Auguste Comte and Positivism* (reprinted Ann Arbor, Mich.: 1961), 1–19, 32–71, 100–24.
49. Georges Canguilhem, *The Normal and the Pathological* (reprinted New York: Zone Books, 1989), 47–89.
50. Hacking, *op.cit.* (ref. 7), 160–9.
51. Canguilhem, *op.cit.* (ref. 49).
52. Comte quoted in Hacking, *op.cit.* (ref. 7), 168.
53. *Ibid..*, 160–9.
54. See also Susan Gross Solomon, 'The Expert and the State in Russian Public Health: Continuities and Changes Across the Revolutionary Divide,' in Dorothy Porter (ed.), *The History of Public Health and the Modern State* (Amsterdam and Atlanta: Rodopi, 1994), 183–223; *idem* and John F. Hutchinson (eds), *Health and Society in Revolutionary Russia* (Bloomington: University of Indiana Press, 1990); Dorothy Porter, 'Changing Disciplines: John Ryle and the Making of Social Medicine in Twentieth-Century Britain,' *History of Science*, 30 (1992), 119–47.

55. Sand, *op.cit.* (ref. 25), 518–20.
56. Originally published as Arthur J.Viseltear, 'Milton C. Winternitz and the Yale Institute of Human Relations: A Brief Chapter in the History of Social Medicine,' *The Yale Journal of Biology and Medicine*, 57 (1984), 869–89.
57. See also Arthur J. Viseltear, 'C. E. A. Winslow and the Early Years of Public Health at Yale, 1915–1925,' *Yale Journal of Biology and Medicine*, 55 (1982), 137–51; *idem,* 'Charles-Edward Amory Winslow, 1877–1957,' *Dictionary of American Biography* (New York: Scribner, 1980), 701–3; Roy Acheson, 'The Epidemiology of Charles-Edward Amory Winslow,' *American Journal of Epidemiology*, 91 (1970), 1–18.
58. Arthur J. Viseltear, 'The Yale Plan of Medical Education: The Early Years,' *Yale Journal of Biology and Medicine*, 59 (1986), 627–48; Roy Acheson and A. M-M. Payne, 'Preventive Medicine at the Yale School of Medicine, 1950–1965,' *Milbank Memorial Fund Quarterly*, 65 (1967), 287–301.
59. Arthur J. Viseltear, 'The Emergence of Pioneering Public Health Education Programmes in the United States,' in Elizabeth Fee and Roy Acheson, *A History of Education in Public Health. Health that Mocks the Doctors' Rules* (Oxford: Oxford Medical Publications, Oxford University Press, 1991),114–54.
60. See Porter, *op.cit.* (ref. 54), 'Changing Disciplines.'
61. For discussion of the planning of the National Health Service see Charles Webster, *Problems of Health Care. The National Health Service Before 1957* (London: Macmillan, 1973); F. Honigsbaum, *Health and Happiness and Security. The Creation of the National Health Service* (London: Routledge, 1989); D. Fox, *Health Policies, Health Politics. The British and American Experiences* (Princeton: Princeton University Press, 1986).
62. See Jane Lewis, *What Price Community Medicine? The Philosophy, Practice and Politics of Public Health Since 1919* (Brighton: Harvester, 1986).
63. See also Dorothy Porter, 'John Ryle: Doctor of Revolution?,' in Dorothy Porter and Roy Porter (eds), *Doctors, Politics and Society: Historical Essays* (Amsterdam: Rodopi, 1993), 229–47.
64. N. T .A. Oswald, 'A Social Health Service Without Doctors,' *Social History of Medicine*, 4 (1991), 295–315.
65. For Haldane see Ronald Clark, *J.B.S. The Life and Work of J.B.S. Haldane* (London: Hodder and Stoughton, 1968); Krisha R. Dronmaraju, *The Life and Work of J.B.S. Haldane, With Special Reference to India* (Aberdeen: Aberdeen University Press, 1985); Gary

Werskey, *The Visible College* (London: Allen Lane, 1978).

66. See Richard A. Soloway, *Demography and Degeneration. Eugenics and the Declining Birthrate in Twentieth-Century Britain* (Chapel Hill: University of North Carolina Press, 1990); Greta Jones, *Social Hygiene in Britain* (London: Croom Helm, 1986); Pauline M.H. Mazumdar, *Eugenics, Human Genetics and Human Failings. The Eugenics Society, its Sources and its Critics in Britain* (London: Routledge, 1992); John Macnicol, 'Eugenics and the Campaign for Voluntary Sterilization in Britain Between the Wars,' *Social History of Medicine*, 2 (1989), 147–70.
67. *Ibid.*, Macnicol.
68. G. R. Searle, 'Eugenics and Politics in Britain in the 1930s,' *Annals of Science*, 35 (1979), 159–69.
69. See also Dorothy Porter, 'Introduction to the Transaction Edition,' to John Ryle, *Changing Disciplines* (New Brunswick: Transaction Books, 1994), xi–xl; *idem, op.cit.* (ref. 54); *idem, op.cit.* (ref. 63).
70. See also Margot Jefferys, 'The Transition from Public Health to Community Medicine: the Evolution and Execution of a Policy for Occupational Transformation,' *Bulletin of the Society for the Social History of Medicine*, 39 (1986), 47–63.
71. See also Margot Jefferys, 'Social Science Teaching in Medical Education: an Overview of the Situation in Great Britain,' in Magdalen Sokolowska *et al.* (eds), *Health, Medicine, Society* (Boston: D. Reidel, 1973); *idem*, 'Serendipity: An Autobiographical Account of the Career of a Medical Sociologist in Britain,' in R. H. Elling and M. Sokolowska (eds), *Medical Sociologists at Work* (New Brunswick: Transactions Press, 1978), 135–61.
72. Philip Abrams, *The Origins of British Sociology: 1834–1914* (Chicago: Chicago University Press, 1968); Martin Bulmer, 'The Development of Sociology and of Empirical Social Research in Britain,' in *idem* (ed.), *Essays on the History of Sociological Research* (Cambridge: Cambridge University Press, 1985). For contrasting institutionalization of social science in the United States see Dorothy Ross, *The Origins of American Social Science* (Cambridge: Cambridge University Press, 1992); Denis Smith, *The Chicago School. A Liberal Critique of Capitalism* (London: Macmillan, 1986).
73. See Ralf Dahrendorf, *LSE. A History of the London School of Economics and Political Science 1895–1995* (Oxford: Oxford University Press, 1995).
74. *Ibid.*, 94–107, 376–80.
75. See also R. H. Elling and M. Sokolowska (eds), *Medical Sociologists at Work* (1978) (ref. 71).
76. See also Smith, *op.cit.* (ref. 72).

77. S. A. Queen and D. M. Mann, *Social Pathology* (New York: Thomas Y. Crowell, 1925).
78. S. A. Queen and J. R. Gruener, *Social Pathology. Obstacles to Social Participation* (New York: Crowell, 1940).
79. John L. Gillin, *Social Pathology* (New York: The Century, 1933).
80. Richard Fuller, *Social Pathology* (New York: 1940).
81. Guy Brown, *Social Pathology. Social and Personal Disorganization* (New York: F. S. Crofts, 1942).
82. Edwin Lemert, *Social Pathology* (New York: McGraw-Hill, 1951).
83. Herbert Blumer, *Symbolic Interactionism* (Berkeley: University of California Press, 1969).
84. See J. Gibbs and M. Erickson, 'Major Developments in the Sociology of Deviance,' *Annual Review of Sociology*, 1 (1975), 21–44.
85. Howard Becker, *Outsiders. Studies in the Sociology of Deviance* (New York: Free Press, 1963); Erving Goffman, *Stigma* (Englewood Cliffs, N.J.: Prentice Hall, 1963); *idem, Asylums* (New York: Doubleday, 1961); *idem, The Presentation of Self in Everyday Life* (Edinburgh: University of Edinburgh Social Scientific Research Centre, 1956).
86. Eliot Freidson, *Futures of Medicine. A Study of the Sociology of Applied Knowledge* (New York: Dodd, Mead, 1970); Talcott Parsons, *The Social System* (New York: Free Press, 1951).
87. M. Stacey with H. Homans, 'The Sociology of Health and Illness: Its Present State, Future Prospects and Potential for Health Research,' *Sociology*,11 (1978), 281–307.
88. Peter L. Berger and Thomas Luckman, *The Social Construction of Reality. A Treatise in the Sociology of Knowledge* (New York: Doubleday, 1966).
89. See also David Armstrong, *The Political Anatomy of the Body* (Cambridge: Cambridge University Press, 1983); *idem*, 'Medical Sociology,' in W. F. Bynum and Roy Porter (eds), *Companion Encyclopedia of the History of Medicine*, 2 vols, (London: Routledge, 1993), Vol. 2 1641–63.
90. George Rosen, *The Specialisation of Medicine: With Particular Reference to Ophthalmology* (New York: Froben, 1944).
91. See also Porter, *op.cit.* (ref. 23).
92. See also Porter, *op.cit.* (ref. 69).
93. Parsons, *op.cit.* (ref. 86).
94. See also David Mechanic, *Medical Sociology: A Selective View* (New York: Free Press, 1968); *idem* and E. H. Volkart, 'Stress, Illness Behaviour and the Sick Role,' *American Sociological Review*, 5 (1961), 51–8.

95. See in particular M. Foucault, *The Birth of the Clinic: An Archeology of Medical Perception* (London: Tavistock, 1973).
96. See Raymond Aron, *Main Currents in Sociological Thought*, 2 Vols (Harmondsworth: Pelican, 1965–9).
97. See also J. A. Clausen and Robert Straus, *Medicine and Society* (Philadelphia: American Academy of Political and Social Science,1963); W. C. Cockeram, *Medical Sociology* (Englewood Cliffs: Prentice-Hall, 1986); Robert Day, 'Toward the Development of a Sociology of Sociology: The Case of Medical Sociology' (Ph.D. thesis, University of Missouri-Columbia, 1981).
98. See also J. Elinson, 'Medical Sociology: Theoretical Underdevelopment and Some Opportunities,' in H. M. Blalock (ed.), *Sociological Theory and Research, a Critical Approach* (New York: Free Press, 1980), 373–81; M. R. Bury, 'Social Constructionism and the Development of Medical Sociology,' *Sociology of Health and Illness*, 8 (1986), 137–69; *idem*, 'Social Constructionism and the Development of Medical Sociology: A Rejoinder to Nicolson and McLaughlin,' *Sociology of Health and Illness*, 9(4) (1987), 439–41.
99. See Bryan S. Turner, *The Body and Society. Explorations in Social Theory* (Oxford: Basil Blackwell, 1984); *idem, Regulating Bodies. Essays in Medical Sociology* (London: Routledge, 1992).
100. Bryan S. Turner, *Medical Power and Social Knowledge* (London: Sage, 1987); *idem*, 'The Practices of Rationality, Michel Foucault, Medical History and Sociological Theory,' in Richard Fardon (ed.), *Power and Knowledge, Anthropological and Sociological Approaches* (Edinburgh: Scottish Academic Press, 1985), 193–213.
101. Robert Straus, 'The Nature of Medical Sociology,' *American Sociological Review*, 22 (1957), 200–4.
102. See Turner, *op.cit.* (ref. 100); also Michael Mann, *The Sources of Social Power*, Vol. 1 (Cambridge: Cambridge University Press, 1986).
103. Raymond Illsley, 'Promotion to Observer Status,' *Social Science and Medicine*, 9 (1975), 63–7.

1

Milton C. Winternitz and the Yale Institute of Human Relations: A Brief Chapter in the History of Social Medicine

Arthur J. Viseltear

'We will never reach the point where we really govern ourselves and master the world until the universities are made centers of communities; until they become civically constructive.'
René Sand
'The Rise of Social Medicine', *Modern Medicine,* 1 (1919), 189

Some time back I published a paper which considered the early years of the Yale Department of Public Health, 1915–25.[1] I now plan to consider a later period, 1925–35, and examine the Institute of Human Relations, a controversial entity comprising the graduate Division of Psychology, the Department of Psychiatry and Mental Hygiene, the Division of Research in Economics, Sociology and Government, and the Division for Research in Child Welfare and Development. At one time or another in its history, the Institute has been referred to as 'a revolutionary advance,' 'an innovative bold step,'[2] on the one hand, and on the other as an interdepartmental stew,[3] an insignificant froth,[4] a concocted scheme far ahead of its time,[5] something analogous to Leacock's gallant warrior 'who mounted his steed and galloped furiously in all directions.'[6]

This episode in the history of the medical school is interesting as it presents all the elements of drama: an intelligent, gifted cast of players, the emergence and implementation of an innovative plan, large sums of money, humour, and disappointment. To tell the story is also to examine the medical school's Dean, Milton C. Winternitz, 'that steam engine in pants', as Yale's President, James Rowland Angell, called him half in jest and half in earnest.[7]

Milton C. Winternitz was certainly someone worth knowing. Liebow and Waters describe him as 'a vital, vivid man, an intense fountainhead of energy, an inexhaustible generator of ideas and constant stimulator of the imagination.'[8] Winslow, a life-long friend, confidant and ally, speaks of Winternitz's 'leaping vision' and of the miracles he achieved,[9] while others, freely acknowledging Winternitz's contributions and accomplishments, describe him less lovingly as a 'martinet,' someone who 'taught by the method of terrorism,' a 'terrible little guy who dissipated the financial resources of the school on impractical schemes.'[10]

Winternitz was elected Dean in 1920, a time when the school faced its most 'disheartening prospects.'[11] The outlook was as unpromising and depressing as could be imagined.[12] But within a few years of his arrival, Winternitz steered the school in a direction leading to excellence and financial stability. His accomplishments were numerous and momentous and a mere listing reveals Winternitz's whole achievement. He first brought the medical school 'into' the university by organizing medical school departments as university departments, opening the medical school and graduate school to each other's students, and assuring that medical faculty met the academic standards of the university; he established the full-time system; found new sources of money for buildings and facilities; designed an 'elastic' curriculum, one that 'liberated' the students' time and was adaptable to individual abilities and needs; established in addition the Department of Psychiatry and Mental Hygiene, a School of Nursing, and institutes devoted to psychobiology and neurology; and, all the while, succeeded in assembling a first-rate faculty that elevated Yale to the front rank of medical institutions in the nation.[13]

Trained at Johns Hopkins, a disciple of William Henry Welch, and a dedicated biomedical scientist, Winternitz's complex personality also revealed a social dimension that is often overlooked when considering the medical school. It is Winternitz's broader, social ideas, which emerged in the 1920s and which found expression and partial fulfilment in the Human Welfare Group and its most controversial and publicized component, the Institute of Human Relations, that are the subject of this chapter.

Part I

The Human Welfare Group, incorporating the schools of nursing and medicine, the New Haven Hospital, New Haven Dispensary, and the Institute of Human Relations,[14] derives from three specific but interrelated roots. The first is the emergence of the social sciences as an academic discipline, including the principle that medicine itself is a socially significant science;[15] the second from the programmes of the

National Research Council established during and immediately following the First World War;[16] and the third from an emerging concept having antecedents in Western Europe which may be called 'Social Medicine,'[17] a concept further embellished in the 1920s by educators as divergent in training and outlook as Lewellys Barker,[18] Richard Cabot,[19] and C.-E. A. Winslow[20] and which appeared as medical school programmes in the 1930s, 1940s and 1950s.[21]

The story of the ravelling of these three roots will take us beyond our allotted time, but, stated simply, emerges as principles established first at the University of Chicago at the turn of the century: that interdisciplinary social scientific research would promote a better understanding of society and help resolve some of its main problems such as waste, inefficiency, and societal and personal maladjustments;[22] that the social sciences would force the university to extend its resources and consider community and societal problems of a practical nature;[23] and that the university, to achieve such ends, would have to break down the barriers erected between departments, programmes and schools.[24]

The First World War, said the Chicago social scientists, resulted from the breakdown of the political and social agencies designed for the controlling of international relations; similarly, they argued, there was an apparent breakdown in human relations. Some form of 'human engineering' was necessary to address and resolve these failures. The question asked was: 'How can society deal with the problems of its own organization so that the proportion of human happiness and satisfying accomplishment may be higher, the proportion of human suffering and failure be lowered?'[25]

This question and ones similar to it were addressed by social scientists in academe, in the Social Science Research Council, and in the National Research Council. The need, wrote Angell, who prior to his Yale appointment had been associated with both the University of Chicago and the National Research Council, was for a more 'penetrating and usable knowledge of human nature.'[26] Given this rather expansive agenda, society itself was the object of study and, as it turned out, Yale was to be its academic locus.

Part II

Why Yale? In the early 1900s, Yale was a quaint and venerable institution, but not as distinguished as it purported to be. George Pierson, writing about the Yale of the 1920s, suggested that its core and justification was not learning or books. You did not come to Yale for an education; instead you came for the real things that Yale offered: contacts, polish and a sense of style.[27] Other than the Sheffield Scientific School, Yale's schools of medicine and law were merely adequate. And it is into this anachronistic and smugly patrician Yale that Angell appeared as its President, Winternitz as its medical school dean, and Robert Maynard Hutchins as Dean of the Law School.

Angell was an outsider who throughout his tenure as President considered himself a 'raw interloper.'[28] He was born in Vermont but spent his formative years in Ann Arbor, where his father served as President of the University of Michigan. Angell attended some of the most prestigious academic institutions in the United States and Europe; was a student or colleague of James, Royce, Dewey, Wundt, Ebbinghaus and Paulsen; advanced 'functionalism' as a school of psychologic thought;[29] served as professor, chairman, Dean and Provost at the University of Chicago, Chairman of the National Research Council and President of the Carnegie Corporation, the holding organization for all the Carnegie philanthropies. Angell was only the second non-Yale man to be appointed a Yale President and, although eminently qualified, he remained for some time a 'stranger,' winning few friends with his proposals to raise academic standards, develop graduate education, and curb the excesses of intercollegiate football. He lacked, what some said with a straight face, the 'patrician arrogance' of the Yale aristocracy and he never touched the university as did his more popular and open predecessor, Arthur Twining Hadley. Nevertheless, Angell's tenure at Yale is considered by most historians as the most important for the future development of modern Yale.[30]

Winternitz we have already met, but Hutchins, whose part in the story is briefest, deserves mention. Whereas Angell was 'distinctly Midwestern,' Winternitz a 'martinet,' Hutchins was the quintessential Yale man. He received his Yale bachelor of arts degree in 1921, was a member of Wolf's Head, the debating team, the Elizabethan Club, Alpha Delta Phi, and was elected Class Orator. Following his commencement, he served for a year as headmaster of a private school in Florida and was then called to succeed the Reverend Anson Phelps Stokes as Secretary of the University, a post he assumed when he was 23 years old. A year later he succeeded Thomas Swan as acting dean of the law school and, two years later, was named its Dean. When Max Mason stepped down as President of the University of Chicago, Hutchins was named his successor, becoming thereby the youngest president of a major university and a legend in the history of American higher education.

How Angell strengthened the university, Winternitz the medical school, and Hutchins the law school is worthy of three distinct papers.

Each worked miracles and the Human Welfare Group and its Institute of Human Relations was to be their greatest success. As it turned out, however, it was the only miracle they were unable to achieve.

Part III

Angell was the prime mover. As chairman of the National Research Council (NRC), he was dedicated to interdisciplinary research and the setting of national agenda, addressing issues such as energy, transportation, forest preservation, and food production. He established NRC divisions of anthropology and psychology, biology and agriculture, chemistry and chemical technology, and industrial relations.[31] At Yale, Angell also fostered the idea of collaborative research. There were societal problems apparent in 'every corner of the corporate body of human society.' It was the university's obligation to address societal issues instead of ignoring them by turning inward. Universities may be slow to change, he said in his Yale inaugural address, but they are still 'plastic.' They are 'living organisms subject to the principles of evolution.'[32]

Angell's university was an integral part of the society it served; it could not be oblivious to the necessities of the social order.

> The university must constantly face, and honestly deal with, the changing obligations which arise from shifting circumstances, and it must be particularly sensitive to those requirements of a given era which are especially urgent, as is in our day a more thorough and scientific understanding of the social and economic fundaments of civilization.[33]

There would always be a place for the 'scholarly recluse' who wished to work in comparative quiet and retirement, he concluded; 'lone scholars of this type must be sheltered and protected.' But:

> large areas of the most significant university work in our day neither invite, nor permit, such complete seclusion, and, while the world may indeed be too much with us, many of the most crucial problems of our generation can only be approached through contacts with the forum and marketplace.[34]

Yale was to be the laboratory to support Angell's thesis.

Angell had his difficulties fitting in, but he was a man of conviction. He allied himself with Wilbur Cross and Edgar Furniss of the graduate school[35] and strengthened the departments of economics, international relations, and history. He sought money to raise academic salaries, raised morale, and drew faculty in each discipline 'across departmental and school boundaries.' He also turned his attention to the medical school and assisted Winternitz in obtaining money from the Commonwealth Fund in support of a programme in mental hygiene, and from the Laura Spellman Rockefeller Memorial Fund for the establishment of an Institute of Psychology, capturing in the process the eminent psychobiologist, Robert Yerkes, and additional monies to enhance the work of Dr Arnold Gesell.

Angell was intrigued by the medical school. He found that much of the research and clinical work of the discrete medical school departments was related, in his word 'correlative,' to university departments. Activities in the departments of paediatrics and public health, the departments of psychology, sociology and government, economics, and anthropology, the divinity school, the school of nursing, and the division of industrial engineering were all relevant to activities in the Institute of Psychology and the Child Guidance Clinic. Even in the law school, Angell noted that Hutchins was initiating plans to bring into the focus of legal studies certain problems of psychology as they affected the law, problems of economics as they related to the field of trade regulation, taxation and finance, and problems of government as these related themselves to legislation, administration and the interpretation of constitutional law. Hutchins, much to Angell's delight, had even begun major programmes of research into the practical procedures of the courts and into the causes and effects of business failures (a study under the direction of William O. Douglas).[36]

But it was Winternitz who captured his imagination. What Winternitz was doing to elevate the medical school was nothing short of miraculous, without parallel in American educational history.[37] And what pleased Angell most was Winternitz's affirmations that medicine was a social science and that the school was not merely a technical institute, but an integral department of the graduate school. Both principles fitted into Angell's grand plan to reform Yale. For example, if the departments of the medical school were university departments, then the same criteria for excellence and scholarly merit would apply to even the clinicians; and if Winternitz believed, as his annual reports revealed, that the Yale medical students would be concerned not only with diseased organs but with the whole man, not only with sickness but with health, not only with biology but with 'man's entire social and economic environment,' then indeed medicine was a social science.

Medicine, wrote Winternitz in 1929, had made great advances.[38] Marvellous methods and instruments for the study of the physical organism had been perfected. But this expansion of knowledge regarding specific functions and organs of the body had necessitated the division of medicine into many specialities. As more and more time had been required for the mastery of a single phase or subspeciality of medicine, 'the physician's time has been diverted increasingly from the patient as an individual.' He continued:

> The old fashioned doctor who was not a specialist, but who knew all about your passion for fishing, who always asked about your son Billy, or who carried away most of your troubles in his little black bag, has become a dim figure on the horizon. It has long been clear that something of the attitude which the old family physician had toward his patients should be restored to medicine.[39]

Medicine was in too many bits and pieces. It was necessary, Winternitz believed, to reassemble the scattered parts of the human organism. Individuals were not only aggregations of cells and organs. They lived in a society. They worked, married, had children. They were happy or unhappy. They encountered disease. They were 'psycho-physical entities,' no part of which could be dealt with satisfactorily except with due consideration of all its functions.

This idea, to regard both the individual and his social environment, to consider both the biological and sociological aspects of life, was not a new concept. Richard Cabot expressed similar ideas in 1909;[40] René Sand did so in 1919,[41] as did C.-E. A. Winslow in 1910, 1920 and 1926,[42] and Lewellys Barker in 1924.[43] But the ideas had not been expressed quite as forcefully as they had been by Winternitz in 1928, nor had they found such receptivity in the financial offices of the private foundations.

Angell, of course, found Winternitz's ideas absolutely in tune with his. The question was how to implement these desultory concepts into a coherent programme. The first need was to gain the support of a number of influential faculty and, accordingly, Winternitz and Hutchins met with colleagues within their respective schools and in other university departments. At these informal occasions, Winternitz and Hutchins pressed forward their ideas with great vigour. Wilbur Cross, then Dean of the graduate school, reminisced about one such meeting during which Winternitz and Hutchins shared their ideas of promoting a synthesis of the biological with the social sciences with such enthusiasm that Cross felt as if he were 'a snowball between two balls of fire which in an instant would consume him.'[44] Cross survived many such meetings and was brought on board, as were

Furniss, Cross's successor, Dodge of Psychology, Dunlop Smith of Industrial Engineering, and Goodrich of Nursing.

As the plans evolved, teaching and research programmes began to emerge. In the Institute, the medical student, for example, was to have an opportunity to consider actual problems of human conduct – such as crime, divorce, unemployment – from legal, social scientific and medical points of view. The medical student was to be working and studying with students of law, religion, economics, government and psychology. In this way, Winternitz believed, the student would constantly meet with the attitude that the individual is at one and the same time a physical, mental and social organism, and that he cannot be properly dealt with unless all of these aspects were considered.[45] 'In his intensity the physician has lost his perspective,' wrote Winternitz:

> ... He has come to be more and more a specialist in a part of the organism rather than a doctor for the whole man. He has become blinded to the psychological and sociological aspects of human well-being overlooking the part played by mind and the environment in reaction with the physical organism.[46]

One of the pamphlets issued by the Institute asked the reader to think of the programme as 'a house,' the 'foundation' of which consists of university sections interested in the fundamental studies of sociology and biology. Resting on this foundation and constituting 'the main floor' of the structure are the applied branches, such as law and medicine, with its affiliated hospital and clinic. On this level contacts with the community are made. The University Health Service would serve as a laboratory for psychological, sociological and economic studies of patients conducted by students and experts of law, medicine and sociology. Information obtained would be taken to 'the upper floors' where, with a broader perspective, sociologists, psychologists, psychiatrists, economists and biologists on the Institute staff would apply themselves to the task of determining the relative significance of the assembled facts.[47]

The hope – 'more than that, the expectation' – was that light would be shed upon societal problems, for example the connections between physical health and family income, mental stability and occupation, crime and the need for recreational facilities, child training and mental growth, economic conditions and divorce, and legal procedures and respect for the law. The pamphlet concluded with a sentence that became an epigram for the entire programme. If the plan were successfully implemented the hope was that it would be possible to bring about a 'readjustment' between the individual and his environment which would lead to 'greater happiness.'[48]

The teaching programme was also described in detail. The proposal was for medical students to be required during their first two years to take a general course in sociology and psychology, a course which would be open to any student in the graduate or professional divisions of the University. Medical students would thus be kept in touch with the problems of life as a whole, a unique proposal, as this was the time in the curriculum usually reserved for the basic sciences.[49]

The sociology course was considered important because it would enable medical students to deal more satisfactorily with human beings when, in their third year, they came into contact with patients for the first time. What Winternitz ultimately proposed and for which he sought funding[50] was a programme in 'Clinical Sociology,' one in which medical students, for example, would be trained in how to be 'social physicians'; that is, how to be 'cognizant of the fundamentals of psychology, biology, and sociology, as well as of traditional legal education.'[51]

Faculty from all disciplines were to pool their resources; students were to be exposed to problems crossing departmental lines; collaborative and interdisciplinary research were to examine societal problems; knowledge was to be correlated. On paper, at least, it was a co-ordinated, unified programme, calling for not only the movement of faculty, but of entire schools and programmes. It was recommended, for example, that the law school be relocated to new facilities adjacent to the medical school on Cedar Street. Similarly, the divinity school, then wishing to move from crowded quarters to a new location, would also be built on property located near to the medical school. Neither school made the move, but consideration of the proposal is an indication of the magnitude of the plan the founders had set forth.[52]

Among the Institute's first publications was a proposal for research revealing the scope of societal concerns to be considered. Research would be undertaken in the following areas: social organization; the structure and function of the central nervous system; prevention of mental illness; the neurological, psychological and biological mechanism of behaviour; the family; race; and demographic patterns in New Haven.[53]

Part IV

Such then was the plan, as set forth in pamphlets, press releases and speeches. Fundraising, as can be imagined, was a full-time activity.

Letters were sent to philanthropic foundations, and Angell and Winternitz, joined by other Yale officers, personally visited the Carnegie Corporation, the Children's Fund of Michigan, the Conrad Hubert Trust, the Falk Foundation, the Julius Rosenwald Fund, the Russell Sage Foundation, the Twentieth Century Fund, and the Josiah Macy Foundation.[54]

A travelling road show was organized, designed to educate the Yale community, alumni and civic groups. Dinners were held in Hartford, Waterbury, Buffalo, Cincinnati, Philadelphia, St Paul, Chicago, New York, Boston and Baltimore. Winternitz, Angell and Yale's treasurer, George Parmly Day, spoke before the Loyal Sons of Yale, The Massachusetts Psychiatric Association, the Mt Sinai Hospital School of Nursing, the Brotherhood of Temple Mishkan Israel in New Haven, and countless Kiwanis Clubs and meetings of the League of Woman Voters.[55]

The speeches presented before those groups conveyed the same themes: knowledge has become compartmentalized; barriers between disciplines must be broken; the goal is to promote human welfare; we are not seeking bits of information but the 'revealed pattern'; our plan is large but not grandiose; we intend to succeed; we need your financial support.[56]

To further assist in the fundraising, an Advisory Committee was established composed of scientists and civic leaders, chaired by William Henry Welch, who could not resist 'the call from his alma mater.'[57] Also agreeing to serve on this committee were Harvey Cushing, Lewellys Barker, Clifford Beers, Franz Boas, George Crile, Surgeon-General Hugh Cumming, John Dewey, Haven Emerson, Harry Emerson Fosdick, Lee Frankel, Charles Evans Hughes, Robert Maynard Hutchins, David Lawrence, Walter Lippmann, William Mayo, Adolf Meyer, Adolf Ochs, Ida Tarbell, Ray Lyman Wilbur, and other notables.[58] Conspicuously absent from this list was Abraham Flexner who, as we shall soon see, was opposed to the Yale plan from the start.

The fundraising campaign was successful, aided in part by the support of the Advisory Committee and specifically by the generous contributions of the Rockefeller Foundation. Seven and a half million dollars was raised[59] and the Institute building constructed adjacent to the existing School of Medicine building located on Cedar Street. A Yale dedication ceremony was planned for 9 May 1931, complete with speeches, tours, a catered luncheon, and even a visit to view the Institute's ape colony. Participating in the ceremonies were Winternitz (who presided at the luncheon), Angell (who presided at the dedication ceremonies held in the inner courtyard of the Institute building), Wilbur Cross, now Governor of Connecticut, Ray Lyman Wilbur, Secretary of the Interior (substituting for President Hoover) and George E. Vincent, former President of the Rockefeller Foundation and a member of the Yale class of 1885.

The speeches were matter-of-fact but conveyed a sense of purpose and optimism. Angell spoke of entering 'upon a new educational procedure' which would exercise a powerful influence throughout Yale and upon educational methods the world over. The Institute, he said, was not a new and separate school; instead it was merely 'an organization devised to bring together into effective voluntary cooperation the various men in the existing University departments of the sciences and arts which bear upon the knowledge and control of human nature and the social order.' Urgent human problems of contemporary life – industrial, medical, economic, legal, educational – would be 'more effectively attacked.' The Institute, he continued, stood more for 'team play than for purely individual endeavor.'[60]

Angell further emphasized the essential nature of the plan. The varied University disciplines have examined only parts of the problem:

> But the understanding of man ... as an active human being involves all ... disciplines ... and cannot be achieved by considering him simply as a body, or as a mind, or as a bank account .... Medicine deals with him when he is ill, law concerns itself with his civil and social behavior, education with his growth and training, theology with his spiritual interests, engineering with his adjustment to the physical environment. But the solution of the more important concrete problems with which men are confronted, either as individuals, or as social groups, almost invariably involves two or more ... sciences or professions. In a given instance poverty may be quite as much a medical problem as an economic one, and even as an enduring social issue it inevitably involves many different factors. Crime has in it psychological, medical, economic, legal, and social elements ... and it cannot be dealt with adequately, either preventively or remedially, without bringing to bear upon it the focalized knowledge and skill involved in a great variety of sciences and professions. And so it is with all the compelling problems of modern life.[61]

The other speakers pursued similar themes. Cross, for example, spoke of 'harmony' and the benefits of 'collective thought'; Wilbur expressed pleasure that the 'vast fund of knowledge,' which has been 'pigeon-holed' would now be collected and better understood;[62] and Vincent waxed eloquent about 'cooperation,' 'physical contiguity,' 'group association,' the 'deepening sense of comradeship,' and the 'stirring adventure.'[63] It was a great day for Yale, and a finer one for Angell and Winternitz. The one cloud on the horizon was the relentless, often acerbic criticism of Abraham Flexner.

Part V

Flexner in 1931 was Director of the Institute of Advanced Study at Princeton and a legendary figure in American higher education. Flexner had great admiration for Winternitz, whom he knew well, and great respect for Angell, whom he knew mainly by reputation. Flexner's contacts with Yale were through George Blumer, Winternitz's predecessor as Dean of the medical school, and then Winternitz himself. Flexner felt possessive about Yale. In 1910, in the famous Report Number Four of the Carnegie Commission, Flexner had written that Yale's medical school was capable of doing better[64] and he saw to it, as the principal officer of the Rockefeller Foundation's General Education Board, that it did. It was Flexner who supported and helped negotiate the closer association of the medical school and the New Haven Hospital and he who favourably reviewed the requests for programmatic assistance.

Winternitz, he believed, was the 'boldest and most enterprising' dean he had encountered and the two remained fast friends, despite their falling out over the Institute, until the 1950s. Winternitz had every right to be upset that Flexner was abandoning them, and Flexner similarly felt put out, acting as does a parent seeing his child go off in pursuit of 'pipedreams.'

Flexner learned of the Institute in Winternitz's 1928–9 Annual Report. He was appalled:

> I read your Annual Report with interest. I wish more fervently than I can express that I could follow and agree with you in the line that you are taking ... but for the life of me I cannot see it, and none of the successive publications which you have [sent] me has as yet cleared the matter up.[65]

Winternitz expressed surprise, and his letters carry the tone of sadness and abandonment.

> I am awfully sorry that you feel as you do .... Rumors come to me from time to time from various sources, and some of them have been quite disturbing, but of course I know that now, as always, you are actuated only in my best interests.[66]

'Why not suspend judgment,' he asked, 'until the Institute is actually in physical existence and the staffs in place?'

Flexner replied:

> I am simply not sympathetic. I share your concern with many things, including the high cost of medical education, and indeed this is one of the reasons why I am sorry to see that you have divided your energy and attention at a critical moment in the history of the enterprise which will forever be associated with your name. Even if we grant that the Institute is worthwhile, I cannot believe it is worth your while at this time, for your hands were full with the medical school and, as you say, you are becoming overburdened .... I am not thinking of the Institute from any personal point of view, yours or mine. But I confess that it worries me as one more of the many instances of vast undertakings commenced without penetrative or sufficient thought and without regard to other obligations of American universities.[67]

All through the early months of 1930, Flexner was revising for publication three lectures on higher education that he had delivered at Oxford in 1928. In 1930 Oxford University Press brought out his *Universities: American, English, German*, in which Flexner documents the errors and follies of some of America's finest universities, not excluding from his sting those in Europe as well.

Flexner's ideal university, unlike that of Angell's, was more in tune with John Henry Newman's.[68] In the ideal university, wrote Flexner, 'we should see to it that in appropriate ways scholars and scientists would be conscious of four concerns: the conservation of knowledge and ideas; the integration of knowledge and ideas; the search for truth; the training of students who will practice and "carry on".' These were the responsibility and sole purpose of a university; anything else, 'however important they may seem, may be carried on elsewhere.' The university was the standard, the home of sweet light and reason. 'There are intellectual standards by which quality may be judged,' he wrote. 'Subjects change; activities change. But ideas and quality abide. The difference between froth and depth, between material and immaterial, between significant and insignificant – that difference persists.'[69]

By the froth, the immaterial and insignificant, Flexner meant institutions such as the teachers' colleges, disciplines such as sociology, and selected 'Institutes' devoted to educational research, international affairs, and child welfare research. The most recent and to Flexner's thinking 'the most incomprehensible development' in the way of an Institute was then taking place at Yale.[70]

Flexner was primarily concerned with the Institute's research agenda and the Institute's assault on 'departmentalization.'[71] Flexner believed that little would ever be learned by studying mental stability and occupations, crime and recreation, or child training and mental growth because these were 'practical tasks,' of 'no concern to a university.'[72] If the research agenda were pure 'folly,' Flexner was totally exasperated by the Institute's organization chart. Why attack departments? he asked. 'Knowledge advances in the first instance only by artificial simplification; departments are set up, not because life in the physical world is simple, but because no progress can be made by observation or experiment unless one's field is circumscribed.'[73]

The Institute, Flexner believed, ignored the necessary individualistic character of genuine thinking. He wondered if 'really first-rate minds,' working in various fields, would be 'artificially or mechanically' brought to cooperate in their studies. 'Science,' he wrote, 'is fundamentally and in the end always an affair of the individual.' Too much planning, too much articulation, he believed, would destroy the freedom of the individual 'upon which in the last resort progress depends.'[74]

At Yale, Flexner's criticisms were taken up by William Harlan Hale, editor of the iconoclastic and forward-thinking *Harkness Hoot.* Hale offered the opinion that the Institute was 'an inter-departmental stew' containing everything from infant psychology and Pauline doctrines of revelations to divorce and thermodynamics:

> No man would dispute the need for a synthesis of human knowledge in a day when specialization is so rampant as is this. But since integrating activities are a matter of the individual, they are to be performed by scholars themselves, not by organizations and grinding machinery. Genuine thinking does not need artificial correlation; that function is itself the unconscious product of clear minds and able workers.[75]

Angell, Winternitz and others protested. Angell was so incensed by Flexner that he told Winternitz that, if Flexner continued to write disparagingly about the Institute, Winternitz should 'write him a very sharp note suggesting that he give his attention more fully to his own affairs.'[76] Even the *Yale Daily News* came to the Institute's defence. In response to Hale's essay, an editorial writer offered a contrasting point of view. 'Yale had not lost sight of the importance of men and become lost in the administration of machinery,' as Hale had suggested:

> The Institute [instead] ... is the empirical philosopher; it is the bygone family practitioner. But before it can diagnose and prescribe, it must know causes and effects. It teaches the successful lawyer, or

the doctor, or the specialist, or the clergyman – in fact anyone interested in human welfare – the essential unity of knowledge.[77]

Part VI

The criticism, however, began to develop an uneasy momentum. Internal dissension and jealousy were present almost from the start. I have just had a meeting with 'the stormy petral,' wrote Angier to Angell; 'Winternitz seems to hold the mistaken idea that, because the Institute building is in his domain, he controls space allocation. He does not.' Angell agreed and so wrote rather bluntly to advise Winternitz.[78]

The unified organizational structure also broke down. At first an Executive Committee of the Institute was formed, composed of Angell, Yale's provost, Charles Seymour, Furniss of the graduate school, Charles Clark (who had succeeded Hutchins as Dean of the School of Law), Winternitz, and Angier of psychology. An Executive Secretary was appointed to handle day-to-day administration, but, when this structure proved unwieldy, Angell reduced the Committee in size and reappointed only Angier, Winternitz and Seymour, adding a well-regarded psychologist, Mark May, as Executive Secretary to oversee discordant points of view.[79]

The publications of the Institute and the media attention were also a cause of concern. Written by the Institute's Director of Publicity, the bulletins and pamphlets had an odd fuzziness about them. What exactly was the Institute about? And how was it to relate to the Human Welfare Group? More important, what was meant by the term 'human happiness,' a phrase which appeared not only in the pamphlets but in the many speeches presented by Angell, Winternitz and others. 'I wish I had interrupted you to ask a definition,' wrote Henry Covell of Rochester. 'I thought I followed you but I'm not sure.'[80] Winternitz was prompted to reply to such queries, especially when they were written by wealthy alumni.

> I am not surprised that you should ask what we mean by 'happiness'. The term, used often by our group, needs defining. I have pondered the question of happiness ever since college and have finally reached a fairly satisfactory conclusion. Happiness may be measured only to the degree to which the psychophysical organism becomes adapted to its environment. The process of adaptation involves an exchange of stimuli between the individual and his environment. Embodied in this definition is recognition of the fact that freedom from dominating physical pain is a prerequisite of happiness ...[81]

Such problems of definition were expected and could be addressed, but other letters found in the Institute's archives reveal that something far more troubling had resulted from the Institute's overly zealous publicity campaign. 'I am in prison on a murder charge,' wrote a man from Kansas. 'I swear I was out of my mind. Can you help me?' Another wrote of his research on breathing, another was concerned about his failing sex drive, while another believed himself an ideal 'case' and sought admission as an inpatient. Even the popular ukulele performer May Singhi Breen wrote to enquire if the Institute could train a mouse for her night-club act![82]

The letters were stashed away in a file and never answered, but two administrative officers of the Institute, Byron Shimp and Henry Lund, realized what their excesses had wrought. Shimp wrote to Angell: 'We must tone down our account of the proposed work.'[83] More important, as many of the newspaper accounts were based on the extemporaneous speeches given by Winternitz and even by Angell himself, Shimp recommended that his office review all drafts of speeches presented on the Institute's behalf. Angell agreed, but the damage had been done. In their endeavour to raise funds for operating expenses and endowment, Institute spokesmen had simply promised more than they could deliver.

There were other problems inherent in the design. Too many of the original Institute faculty brought their own research with them and never gave a thought to collaborating, except to present, at most, a seminar. As a result eighty per cent of the monies raised by Institute-funded projects were initiated by individuals and not collaborative groups.[84] Despite geographic proximity and professed interest, the 'larger pattern' never emerged.

Many of these issues were addressed in 1930 when Mark May took over as Executive Director. May found a distinguished faculty, but observed that most were working, Gesell, for example, 'in splendid isolation as far as the rest of the Institute is concerned.' Funds were always in short supply, especially during the Depression years, but what about the funds that had been raised? Could funds be used as 'the impetus for cooperative work?' 'Does being a member of the Institute mean that all problems will perforce be of an interdisciplinary nature?' May asked. And a final concern: 'How are we to conserve those elements of individual freedom, initiative, inventiveness, and imagination, which are regarded as essential in scientific discovery, and at the same time follow a formal program?[85]'

The problem was that no one had thought through more than superficially the mechanisms by which mere geographic proximity would work its magic. Moreover, no one wished to abrogate the academic right to work on problems that were of personal interest only. When Angell was Chairman of the National Research Council he was able to establish a bureaucratic plan for research owing to the exigencies of the First World War, but once the war ended the scientists resisted administrative control of their research. Jacques Loeb in 1920, for example, wrote to Ernest Rutherford that National Research Council staff were reviewing every research proposal to root out duplication of effort, or to establish a policy of targeted research. Such information was to be provided 'voluntarily,' wrote Loeb, 'but given a good American political machine, and the money to back it with, and I should like to see which young men will dare to stand up against it.'[86] Bureaucracy would ruin science and many believed that this would happen at Yale.

Part VII

And what of Winternitz and the medical school? What went wrong with the ideas he had set forth in 1928? Yale, he wrote in his Annual Report, is not interested in training 'doctor-technicians;' here we favour 'the development of physicians and humanitarians.'[87] At Yale there was to be a 'fostering of interrelationships of the many specialties and sciences upon which medicine depends.' For too long, he wrote, our students' attention has been 'concentrated on fragments of the biological organism.' We are 'endangering the broader aspects of medicine.' The Yale plan calls for an 'integration of Knowledge.' Yale's 'pure objective' is nothing less than 'the well-being of man.'[88] Winslow in 1935 summarized the essence of Winternitz's theses as follows: Medicine is a social science; medicine should deal with the welfare of the patient through his whole life and should visualize the promotion of health as a positive ideal; medicine should be concerned with the whole man as a human personality, with a mind and emotions as well as the heart and lungs.[89]

The entire plan signified that the time had come for a 'new synthesis inspired by a new humanism.'[90] It was perhaps a 'synthetic humanism'[91] to be sure, but fundamental principles were being set forth at Yale about the roles in society of both medicine and the university. The great advances in the adaptation of the sciences to diagnosis and therapy leading to specialization had led to the narrowing of physicians' interests. The patient had been reduced to mere bits and pieces. Societal influences, such as housing, employment, poverty, bankruptcy, class status, all had been pushed to one side. Public health and preventive medicine in the medical curriculum suffered the worst fate of all, indifference. And this was not just true of the medical school. University departments had also turned inward. Those programmes that did attempt interdisciplinary work, venturing across the impenetrable membranes that contained cognate disciplines, were ridiculed for abandoning the main objectives of higher education. René Sand and others argued just the opposite. Universities, Sand wrote in 1919, should be 'civically constructive.'[92] Angell, with a pedigree rooted in the University of Chicago, 'functionalism' and the National Research Council, agreed, and went a step further, arguing that the survival of the University was dependent upon the recognition of the peculiar exigencies of the present and needs of the future.[93] The Human Welfare Group and its Institute of Human Relations were looking for the revealed pattern, a 'fresh synthesis,'[94] in Mark van Doren's felicitous phrase, 'the connectedness of things.'[95]

Winternitz set the programme in motion, but confronted insurmountable problems in his parent institution. He was respected for his brilliance and dynamism, but many of the allies he had assembled soon deserted him, considering his policies autocratic and misguided. Rumblings in the Board of Permanent Officers, the governing body of the medical school composed of the senior faculty, were evident early in his first term. Implementing the full-time system opened many wounds that never healed. Faculty found it necessary to appeal directly to the President and a palace revolt was barely averted when Winternitz, counting the votes, was forced to establish a number of standing committees, the principal recommendation of a governance committee that had been appointed to review administrative procedures but, as everyone knew, took as their charge the design of a plan to decentralize authority.[96]

Winslow and a few others remained loyal. When in 1929 Winternitz had been reappointed, Winslow wrote him a note of congratulations. Winternitz replied:

> When I got back from St. Paul last night there were two letters, one from the University and the other from you, both conveying my reappointment. The first was a statement like a newspaper notice for a birth or a death and then your kind note which took the bitter taste out of my mouth. Do you know it is, I think, the only expression of opinion I have had from any of our B.P.O. not only about this but about anything that has ever happened in this year at Yale. And so it touched me the more deeply. After all we are children and like to get a pat on the back like the rest occasionally.[97]

Winslow's friendship and loyal support was especially expressed in an inspiring address he presented on the occasion of Winternitz's 'retirement.' It was a bitter-sweet occasion because it signalled not a retirement but a defeat and abrupt ouster. It is evident that Winternitz knew he would not be reappointed to another term in 1934, but he resisted the inevitable for some time. The BPO, composed of many faculty whom he himself had brought to Yale and nurtured, had simply grown weary of his policies and continued bold schemes and refused to vote in favour of reappointment. Winternitz appealed to Angell, enquiring about the possibility of a Presidential or Corporation reappointment.[98] Angell, however, also counting the votes, refused to go over the head of the medical school's senior faculty and Winternitz finally accepted reality. No one mentioned these events and referred to the occasion only as Winternitz's 'retirement,' which is why Winslow's eloquent testimonial address delivered on Alumni Day, 17 June 1935, was so moving.[99] Winternitz wrote immediately to Winslow:

> Dear Charlie:
> What a man! The evening is over as is the night and I am still trembling. Nothing but the most loyal, most sincere devotion could inspire a man as you were inspired yesterday. The hours you must have labored in the preparation of the masterful address – enough in itself – is as nothing compared to the power, the feeling, the magnificence of your delivery. It will live all my life as a burning torch of friendship such as few men have the privilege of knowing. I am deeply grateful.[100]

Part VIII

Winternitz gave many more years of devoted service to Yale,[101] but he was mortally wounded by the events of 1935. Had he never entertained the idea for the Institute would he have been more successful? Probably not. John F. Fulton, one of Winternitz's most important and famous medical school and Institute appointments, and a loyal friend, probably said it best. In a letter to C. N. H. Long written in 1942 about Winternitz's plan for an 'atypical growth program,' which 'Winter had developed in his mind's eye and [had] much to be said for it,' Fulton reminded Long 'not to forget' Winternitz's plans for the Institute of Human Relations 'and the fact that Winter finds it a constitutional necessity to draw up broadly conceived over-all programs about once a month.'[102] Winternitz, to many, had simply moved too fast. The ideas he expressed in the 1920s and 1930s were simply too diffuse, bold and idealistic to resist the scientific and technological imperatives of modern medicine. In each of the Yale basic science and clinical departments great advances were taking place in neurophysiology, pharmacology, infectious diseases, endocrinology, metabolism, clinical trials, and surgical and medical interventions and innovations. These were the subjects that captured the interest of the young medical students. Winslow, since his arrival at Yale in 1915, had tried to infuse a 'pervasive preventive spirit' into the curriculum and, in part, he was successful; but not a single medical student took the opportunity, which the Yale curriculum offered, to enter coursework leading to a joint degree in public health.[103] What soon mattered in the Winternitz years, despite the Institute and its champions, was not prevention but cure; not the community but the patient; not health but sickness – each a negation of the principles upon which the Institute had been founded.

And this takes us to the present. What is Winternitz's and the Institute's legacy? Not surprisingly, as with most things, the spores of the ideas originally set forth are finding fertile soil. The principles espoused by Winternitz and his colleagues, for example, are similar to the principles upon which Yale's Institution for Social and Policy Studies has been based;[104] they are the rationale behind interdisciplinary cooperation and integrated research, as found, for example, in Yale's Comprehensive Cancer Center and Whitney Humanities Center;[105] they are the principles which are now reappearing in today's call for curricular revisions designed to produce more broadly and humanistically educated physicians;[106] they appear again in academic speeches at Yale and elsewhere, as in Michael Sovern's Columbia University inaugural presidential address, in which he calls for 'a grand synthesis' in education;[107] and they form the basis for our contemporary health-care 'composites' known as academic health centres.[108]

Seen from our present perspective, the plans of Winternitz, Angell, Hutchins and their colleagues were not a negation of science and speciality training, for each recognized the importance and need for specialists in society, but were rather an attempt to place the powerful engine of science on a more humanistic and socially oriented roadbed, to reverse a tendency in medicine to the particular at the expense of the universal, and to harness the creative energies of the university on behalf of society.

Acknowledgement

The original publication of this essay was supported in part by NIH grant LM 03746 from the National Library of Medicine.

Notes

1. Viseltear, A. J., 'C-E A Winslow and the Early Years of Public Health at Yale, 1915–1925,' *Yale J Biol Med,* 55 (1982), 137–51.
2. Harvard Alumni Bulletin, 'Yale's New Institute,' *Yale Alumni Weekly* (15 March 1929), 730.
3. Hale, W. H., 'The Madness at New Haven,' *Harkness Hoot,* 1 (1931), 9–22.
4. Flexner, A., *Universities: American, English, German* (New York: Oxford University Press, 1930), 43.
5. Paul, J. R., 'Dean Winternitz and the Rebirth of the Yale Medical School in the 1920's,' *Yale J Biol Med,* 43 (1970),110–19.
6. Orton, W., 'Synthetic Humanism at Yale,' *Yale Alumni Weekly* (5 April 1929), 826.
7. Pierson G. W., *Yale: The University College, 1921–1937* (New Haven: Yale University Press, 1955), 260.
8. Liebow, A. A. and Waters, L. L., 'Milton Charles Winternitz, February 19, 1885–October 3, 1959,' *Yale J Biol Med,* 32 (1959), 143–72.
9. Winslow, C.-E. A., *Dean Winternitz and the Yale School of Medicine; Address Delivered Before the Association of Yale Alumni in Medicine on 17 June 1935* (New Haven: Yale University Press, 1935), 17.
10. Paul, *op. cit.* (ref. 5).
11. Angell, J. R., *Report of the President, 1934–1935* (New Haven: Yale University, 1935), 15.
12. *Ibid.*, 15; see also *The Past, Present and Future of the Yale University School of Medicine ...* (New Haven: Printed for the University, 1922), 5–8.
13. See, for example, Winternitz, M. C., 'Medical Education at Yale University: A Summary of Its Progress in Recent Years,' *Yale Alumni Weekly* (29 January 1932), 345–7. See also Winternitz, M.C., 'The Graduate Plan in Medical Education,' *Journal of the Association of American Medical Colleges* 2 (1927), 208–13, and Stockard, C.R., 'Medical Education and the Yale Announcement,' *JAMA,* 86 (1926), 1508–11.
14. *The Human Welfare Group, New Haven, Connecticut; For the Promotion of Health, Physical and Mental, Individual and Social* (New Haven: General Hospital Society, Yale University, 1929).
15. Winternitz, M. C., 'Medicine as a Social Science,' in L. D. White (ed.) *The New Social Science* (Chicago: University of Chicago Press, 1930), 40–5.
16. See Angell, J. R., 'The National Research Council,' in R. M. Yerkes (ed.), *The New World of Science; Its Development During the War,* (New York: Century Co., 1920), 417–38; see also Hale, G. E.,

'The Purpose of the National Research Council,' *Bull National Research Council,* 1 (1919), 1–7; and Angell, J.R., 'The Organization of Research,' *Scientific Monthly,* 11 (1920), 26–42.

17. Rosen, G., 'What is Social Medicine?,' *Bull Hist Med,* 21 (1947), 674–733.
18. Barker, L. F., 'The Social Significance of Medicine,' *Med J and Record,* 120 (1924), 53–6.
19. Cabot, R. C., *Social Service and the Art of Healing* (New York: Dodd, Mead and Co., 1931).
20. Winslow, C.-E. A., 'The Untilled Fields of Public Health,' *Modern Medicine,* 2 (1920), 6–7.
21. See, for example, Galdston, I., *Social Medicine; Its Derivation and Objectives* (New York: Commonwealth Fund, 1949).
22. See, for example, Ogburn, W. F. and Goldenweiser, A., *The Social Sciences and Their Interrelations* (New York: Houghton Mifflin Co., 1927).
23. Seligman, E. R. A., 'What are the Social Sciences?,' in E. R. A. Seligman and A. Johnson (eds) *Encyclopedia of the Social Sciences,* (New York: Macmillan & Co., 1930), Vol. 1, 3–7.
24. Ogburn, W. F. and Goldenweiser, A., 'The Field of the Social Sciences,' in *The Social Sciences* (ref. 22), 1–9.
25. Angell, J. R., 'Yale's Institute of Human Relations,' reprinted from *The Yale Alumni Weekly* (19 April 1929), 4.
26. *Ibid.*
27. Quoted by Pierson, *op. cit.* (ref. 7), 106.
28. Angell, J. R., 'James Rowland Angell,' in C. Murchison (ed.), *A History of Psychology in Autobiography,* (Worcester: Clark University Press, 1936), III, 1–38; see also Miles, W., 'James Rowland Angell, 1869–1949; Psychologist-Educator,' *Science,* 110 (1949), 1–4.
29. Angell, J. R., 'The Province of Functional Psychology,' *Psychological Review,* 14 (1907), 61–91.
30. See Pierson, *op. cit.* (ref. 7), 164–89, and Kelley, B. M., *Yale; A History* (New Haven: Yale University Press, 1974), 369–92. Kelley entitles his chapter 'James Rowland Angell and the Triumph of the University.' 'Patrician arrogance' was a phrase coined by Lucius Beebe in an article entitled, 'Childe Rowland of Yale,' in the *New York Herald Tribune,* 11 January 1931.
31. Angell, J. R., 'The National Research Council' (ref. 16).
32. Angell, J. R., 'Inaugural Address,' in Angell, J. R., *American Education; Addresses and Articles.* (New Haven: Yale University Press, 1937), 6.
33. Angell, J. R., 'Aims of the University,' in *ibid.,* 101.
34. *Ibid.,* 101–2.

35. Furniss, E. S., *The Graduate School of Yale; A Brief History* (New Haven: printed for the Graduate School, 1965), 111–13.
36. Hutchins, R. M., 'Law and the New Institute,' *Yale Alumni Weekly* (8 March 1929), 697–8.
37. Angell, *op. cit.* (ref. 11), 15; see also James Rowland Angell to George Parmly Day, 5 March 1927, Papers of the Provost, Yale University, 43, 427.
38. Winternitz, M. C., 'Medicine and the Human Welfare Group,' *The Human Welfare Group at New Haven; A Series of Informal Discussions of a New Educational Project,* Number II, 1929 (Rockefeller Archives Center, 1.4.636).
39. *Ibid.*
40. Cabot, *op. cit.* (ref. 19). Cabot's *Social Service and the Art of Healing* was first published in 1909 and reprinted in 1928 and 1931. See also Warbasse, J. P., *Medical Sociology* (New York: D. Appleton and Co., 1909).
41 Sand, R., 'The Rise of Social Medicine,' *Modern Medicine,* 1 (1919), 189–91.
42. Winslow, *op. cit.* (ref. 20). See also Winslow's American Public Health Association Presidential Address: 'Public Health at the Crossroads,' *American Journal of Public Health,* 15 (1926), 1075–85.
43. Barker, *op. cit.* (ref. 18). See also Barker, L. F., 'Comments on Health and Life, and on the Broadening Conceptions of the Tasks of Practicing Physicians,' *Annals of Clinical Medicine,* 4 (1926), 525–34.
44. Cross, W. L., *Connecticut Yankee; An Autobiography* (New Haven: Yale University Press, 1943), 181.
45. Winternitz, M. C., 'Medical Education at Yale University; A Summary of its Progress in Recent Years,' *Yale Alumni Weekly* (29 January 1932), 347.
46. Winternitz, M. C., 'The Human Welfare Group,' *Yale Alumni Weekly* (7 March 1930), 686.
47. *Yale Proposes to Study Man* (New Haven: The Human Welfare Group, 1929), 10–12.
48. *Ibid.*, 12–13.
49. *Ibid.*, 16–17.
50. *Ibid.*, 17–18. See also Milton C. Winternitz to Michael M. Davis, 14 December 1931, and Davis to Winternitz, 28 December 1931 (Yale School of Medicine, Dean's Files, Box 2). The Winternitz–Davis correspondence extends for a number of years. Davis was working as a principal adviser to the Julius Rosenwald Fund and, despite his interest in 'clinical sociology' and the application of the social sciences to medicine, Davis was unable to convince the Fund to support Winternitz's proposals. See Davis's 'Social Medicine as a Field for Social

Research,' *American Journal of Sociology*, 44 (1938), 273–9. See also Winternitz to Rosenwald, 22 October 1931 (Yale School of Medicine, Dean's Files, Box 2). The 'Dean's Files' have been deposited in Manuscripts and Archives, Yale University Library.

51. Winternitz, M. C., *Report of the Dean of the School of Medicine ... 1930–1931*, 50–1.
52. Furniss, *op. cit.* (ref. 35), 54–6. See also John Farwell to Charles Seymour, 5 July 1928, Papers of the Provost, Yale University, 36, 360, and L. A. Weigle to M. C. Winternitz, 9 January 1929, *ibid.*
53. See *Report to the National Advisory Committee of the Human Welfare Group* (New Haven: March 1930), 15–27.
54. For information about Institute fundraising activities, see the papers of James Rowland Angell, 110, 1121. The Angell Papers have been deposited in Manuscripts and Archives, Yale University Library. See also Byron W. Shimp to George Parmly Day, 12 October 1931 (Yale School of Medicine, Dean's Files, II, 6).
55. Angell Papers, 110, 1121.
56. The speeches may be found in Angell Papers, *op. cit.* (ref. 55). Additional speeches may be found in Yale Research Group 27, II, 5–6.
57. William Henry Welch to James Rowland Angell, 4 February 1929 (Angell Papers, 110, 1122). See also Winternitz to Welch, 9 February 1929 (Papers of William Henry Welch, Box 62). The Welch papers have been deposited in the Alan M. Chesney Medical Archives, Johns Hopkins Medical Institutions, Baltimore, Maryland.
58. Papers relating to the National Advisory Committee may be found in Yale Research Group 27, II, 5–6. See also *Report to the National Advisory Committee of the Human Welfare Group* (New Haven: March 1930).
59. 'The Yale Institute of Human Relations Established for the Study of Man's Behavior with Gifts Representing a Capital of $7,500,000,' *Yale Alumni Weekly* (15 February 1929), 597–8.
60. 'President Angell's Speech,' *Addresses Delivered at the Dedication of the Institute of Human Relations, Yale University, May 9, 1931*, 1 (Angell Papers, 108, 1103).
61. *Ibid.*, 1–2.
62. 'Address of Governor Wilbur L. Cross,' *ibid.*, 2.
63. *Ibid.*, 3–4.
64. Flexner, A., *Medical Education in the United States and Canada ... Bulletin Number Four* (New York: Carnegie Foundation for the Advancement of Teaching, 1910), 199–200.
65. Abraham Flexner to Milton C. Winternitz, 8 January 1930 (Papers of Abraham Flexner, Box 15). The Flexner Papers have been deposited in the Library of Congress.

66. Milton C. Winternitz to Abraham Flexner, 13 January 1930, *ibid.*
67. Abraham Flexner to Milton C. Winternitz, 14 January 1930, *ibid.*
68. Newman, J. H., *The Idea of a University,* 1852. For a contrasting view see Huxley, T. H., *Science and Culture,* (London: Macmillan, 1881). See also Kerr, C., *The Uses of the University* (Cambridge, Mass.: Harvard University Press, 1963).
69. Flexner, *op. cit.* (ref. 4), 43.
70. *Ibid.*, 112.
71. *Ibid.*, 114.
72. *Ibid.*, 113.
73. *Ibid.*, 114.
74. *Ibid.*, 119.
75. Hale, *op. cit.* (ref. 3), 13.
76. James Rowland Angell to Milton C. Winternitz, 15 April 1930 (Yale School of Medicine, Dean's Files, I).
77. 'The Institute and Mr. Hale,' *Yale Daily News,* 9 May 1931.
78. Roswell P. Angier to James Rowland Angell, 29 October 1929 (Angell Papers, 109, 1109). See also Angell to Winternitz, 5 June 1930, and Winternitz to Angell, 7 June 1930 (Angell Papers, 108, 1093).
79. Corporation Secretary to James R. Angell, 12 December 1931 (Provost's Files, Yale University, 36, 359).
80. Henry H. Covell to Milton C. Winternitz, 21 March 1932 (Yale School of Medicine, Dean's Files, I, 5).
81. Milton C. Winternitz to Henry H. Covell, 9 January 1930, *ibid.*
82. These letters are found in the Papers of the Institute of Human Relations, 37–V, II,10, 69. The Papers have been deposited in Manuscripts and Archives, Yale University Library.
83. Byron Shimp to James Rowland Angell, 11 October 1929. See also Edgar S. Furniss to Milton C. Winternitz, 30 January 1930 (Angell Papers, 110, 1121); Roswell P. Angier to Milton C. Winternitz, *ibid.*; James Rowland Angell to Harold Lund, 27 March 1931, *ibid.*; and Agenda for Institute of Human Relations Meeting, Executive Committee, 29 October 1929 (Provost's Papers, Yale University, 35, 360).
84. Mark May to James Rowland Angell, 28 October 1932, 1 (Angell Papers, 109, 1109).
85. *Ibid.*, 13–14.
86. Jacques Loeb to Ernest Rutherford, 31 August 1920. Cited in Reingold, N. and Reingold, I. H., *Science in America; A Documentary History, 1900–1939* (Chicago: University of Chicago Press, 1981), 307–8.
87. Winternitz, M. C., *Report of … [the] Dean, 1928–1929,* 13.
88. *Ibid.*

89. Winslow, *op. cit.* (ref. 9), 12–13.
90. Winslow, C.-E. A., 'Public Health and the Human Welfare Group,' *The Human Welfare Group at New Haven; A Series of Informal Discussions of a New Educational Project,* Number VII, 1930 (Rockefeller Archives Center, 1.4.636).
91. Orton, *op. cit.* (ref. 6).
92. Sand, *op. cit.* (ref. 41), 189.
93. Angell, *op. cit.* (ref. 32), 6.
94. Angell, J. R., 'Specialization and the Broader Needs of our Time,' *op. cit.* (ref. 32), 75.
95. Van Doren, M., *Liberal Education* (New York: Henry Holt and Co., 1943), 115.
96. See, especially, *Prudential Committee Minutes,* Yale School of Medicine, 9 December 1932, and *Minutes of the Board of Permanent Officers,* 11 October 1932.
97. Milton C. Winternitz to C.-E. A. Winslow, 14 February 1929 (Charles-Edward Amory Winslow Papers, I, 32, 825). The Winslow Papers have been deposited in Manuscripts and Archives, Yale University Library.
98. See *Prudential Committee Minutes,* Yale School of Medicine, 21 November 1934; *Minutes of Board of Permanent Officers,* 12 December, 1934, and 19 December 1934, and Milton C. Winternitz to James Rowland Angell, 11 April 1935 (Yale School of Medicine, Dean's Files, I, 'Angell (2)').
99. Winslow, *op. cit.* (ref. 6).
100. Milton C. Winternitz to C.-E. A. Winslow, 18 June 1935 (Winslow Papers, I, 32, 827).
101. See, for example, Liebow and Waters, *op. cit.* (ref. 8).
102. John F. Fulton to C. N. H. Long, 20 May 1943 (John F. Fulton Papers). The Fulton Papers have been deposited in Manuscripts and Archives, Yale University Library.
103. See Viseltear, *op. cit.* (ref. 1), 146. For a review of Yale biomedical science, see Liebow, A. A., 'Medical Research at Yale in the Twentieth Century,' *Yale J Biol Med* 33, 193–211, 1960.
104. See Institution for Social and Policy Studies' Bulletins and *A Proposal for the Creation of an Institute of Social Science,* Yale University, 17 April 1968.
105. See Giamatti, A. B., *Introductory Remarks on the Occasion of the Inauguration of the Whitney Humanities Center,* Yale University, 4 February, 1981, 2.
106. See, for example, Bok, D., *President's Report* [to the Board of Overseers of Harvard University], *1982–83,* March 1984.

107. Sovern, M. I., *Inaugural Address,* Columbia University, 28 September 1980.
108. See, for example, Roger, D., *American Medicine; Challenge for the 1980s.* (Cambridge, Mass.: Ballinger Publishing Company, 1978), and Sheps, C. G. and Lewis I. J.: *The Sick Citadel; The American Academic Medical Center and the Public Interest.* (Cambridge, Mass.: Oelgeschlager, Gunn & Hain, 1983).

2

Training Doctors for the National Health Service: Social Medicine, Medical Education and the GMC 1936–48

Nigel Oswald

In this chapter I intend to explore a particular aspect of the preparation for the introduction of the National Health Service (NHS). My argument is that the approach to medical planning and medical care called 'social medicine' informed an active debate about the way doctors, especially general practitioners (GPs), should practise. In the context of the proposals to introduce the NHS the ideas of social medicine proponents gained in importance, and a serious attempt was made to embed the ideas of social medicine firmly within the medical curriculum. This was necessary in order to train doctors for the work that would be required of them if the ideals of the NHS were to be achieved.

In the event the campaign to reorientate medical education, though vigorous, was unsuccessful. The basis of the medical service in the United Kingdom was fundamentally altered by the introduction of the NHS, but medical training changed very little. The mismatch between training and practice has never been resolved, and constitutes one of the reasons why NHS activity has made so little impact on the main areas of preventable and chronic illness.

It may seem self-evident to many reading this chapter that the clinical aspects of human illness are inextricably linked with their social aspects. It is worth remembering that this is not self-evident to all, or even most, doctors. The reason for this is that what is perceived by both doctors and patients as the most significant parts of a clinical doctor's life occur face to face, when one doctor is communicating with one patient. In such an interview the patient and their problem is separated from the patient's normal context, and in particular from the needs or difficulties of others. Usually there is a 'problem' to be solved which has an immediacy which gives it precedence over all other considerations. Where this patient's problem fits into the spectrum of similar problems is a secondary matter which may, by common consent, receive scant attention from either patient or doctor. It requires a major reorientation of priorities on both sides if people and their doctors are going to take seriously the issues of health promotion and disease prevention. It was just this reorientation which the proponents of social medicine were keen to introduce, and the remainder of this chapter attempts to sketch a background to their attempt and to explain its failure.

What was the Meaning of 'Social Medicine?'

In the period with which I am concerned the term 'social medicine' in the United Kingdom represented the spectrum of views of a disparate group of doctors who were preoccupied with the role which doctors might fulfil in realizing 'progressive' change in society. Proponents embarked on a programme to introduce change, but so rapid was the rise to prominence and subsequent fall of 'social medicine' that it was never fully articulated or tested. However, there were twin foundations to the argument: the first was the affirmation that the interest of individuals and of the society to which they belonged coincided in maximizing health. The second was that it was impossible to separate the medical activities involved in curing the sick from activities designed to promote health. Both elements were essential and, this being the case, both were the business of doctors and the educators of doctors. The Goodenough Committee,[1] which took the arguments of social medicine as central to its remit, used this definition:

> As used by us the term 'social medicine' includes the more restricted, though very important, subject of disease prevention. It also signifies a particular conception of Medicine; a conception that regards the promotion of health as a primary duty of the doctor, that pays heed to man's social environment and heredity as they affect health, and that recognises that personal problems of health and sickness may have communal as well as individual aspects.

It is thus easy to see how issues of equity, resources, prevention and large-scale planning all featured largely in the statements about social medicine.

Why did we get a National Health Service?

I introduce this question not to go over ground comprehensively covered by others but because of the multiple connections between the positive proposals of the social medicine lobby and the perceived deficiencies of the medical service in the late 1930s. Individuals were writing and speaking about a 'social' perspective on medical services before there were firm proposals for a national health service. However, the development of these ideas was undoubtedly accelerated by the events of the Second World War and the re-evaluations which accompanied them. The period between 1940 and 1945 saw a rapid increase in the attention paid to social medicine proponents. This was followed by an even more rapid waning of their power, even though the NHS, which should have been the embodiment of their ideas, was placed irrevocably on the political agenda during the period of their ascendancy. The medical service in the UK in the late 1930s was inadequate in quality and organization, was grossly unevenly distributed, racked by rivalry and competition, in constant financial crisis and unsuitable for any kind of large-scale planning.[2,3] The social medicine programme addressed each of these deficiencies: the creation of an equitable, high-quality, planned national service, supported by Exchequer funds, would be in the interest of both society and individuals, and equates with the 'Visions of Utopia' referred to by Webster.[4] At the same time the bringing together of the interests of general practitioners and hospital-based specialists through the integration of preventive and curative services not only suggested a way of encouraging progressive change, but also carried implications for the way a doctor should be educated. Indeed it suggested that there was a large aspect of a doctor's work which had been shamefully neglected and which should now be given proper recognition. This neglected area was in the promotion of health among individuals and in communities. Doctors were used to responsibility only for individuals who were in the role of patient and the idea that they might accept an obligation to whole communities involved a radical change in attitude and in the organization of medical services.

The roots of this thinking can be traced back to at least the end of the nineteenth century. The poor physical health of the soldiers conscripted for the Boer War was a shock to those who were aware of it. In 1906 George Newman, Medical Officer of Health in Finchley, wrote of the death of young children in his Borough (165 per 1000 live births) and chose to call his book 'Infant Mortality: a

Social Problem.'[5] A little later the Royal Commission on the Poor Law reported,[6] and in their subsequent book Sidney and Beatrice Webb drew attention to the preventable aspects of the ill-health which brought so many to the misery of the workhouse.[7]

The First World War again gave prominence to the vital importance of a fit population which could reproduce easily stock which was healthy and resilient. In the aftermath of the war the necessity for a Ministry to oversee health matters was acknowledged and George Newman, who had become Chief Medical Officer in the Ministry of Education, was installed as the first Chief Medical Officer. In one of the Ministry's first initiatives he entrusted to Sir Bertrand Dawson the Chairmanship of a Consultative Council on Medical and Allied Services, and it was in the interim (and only) Report of this Council[8] that the inseparability of curative and preventive services was articulated.[9] Dawson stated:

> Preventive and curative medicine cannot be separated on any sound principle, and in any scheme of medical services must be brought together in close co-ordination....They must both likewise be brought together within the sphere of the general practitioner, whose duties should embrace the work of communal as well as individual medicine.

This was the first expression of an idea which was refined as the programme for social medicine developed.

As an expression of this interdependence Dawson proposed the setting up of health centres which would provide facilities ranging from welfare services to in-patient beds, and that both general practitioners and specialists should practise in them. This did not prove a fruitful proposal because of interprofessional resistances and anxieties. However, during the next decade the Peckham experiment, centred on the Pioneer Health Centre, was established.[10,11] Here principles of self-help were brought together with a philosophy of positive health to give, perhaps, a glimpse of what 'health for all' might mean. Peckham was an isolated example which did not lead to widespread imitation, but it had a strong appeal.

Meanwhile, the development of local authority welfare services in, for example, maternity and child welfare, coupled with changes in medical technology which required increasingly sophisticated hospital provision, resulted in a gradually rising status for the Municipal Hospitals. Issues such as hospital co-ordination were addressed in the 1929 Local Government Act. At the same time individuals were considering social objectives in their thoughts about the medical service. It is time to trace the contribution of some of these people. Newman and Dawson remained active: Newman continued in the post of Chief Medical Officer until 1935. Dawson became an elder statesman, elevated to the House of Lords and, in spite of his age, able to speak strongly in favour of the Beveridge proposals in 1942,[12] and to find himself put forward once more as the President of the BMA in 1943. Others were prominent in the debate, and I shall focus on the activities of five people: Sir Farquhar Buzzard, Regius Professor of Physic at Oxford; Sir Wilson Jameson, Professor of Public Health at the London School of Hygiene and Tropical Medicine and, from 1940, Chief Medical Officer at the Ministry of Health; Professor John Ryle, Regius Professor of Physic in Cambridge, appointed the first-ever Professor of Social Medicine in Oxford in 1943; Dame Janet Vaughan, at that time a younger Fellow of the Royal College of Physicians (RCP), and Sir James Spence, Professor of Paediatrics in Newcastle.

This is a disparate group, but it is their activities and the interaction of their interests which are central to my claim that there was an active campaign for social medicine among influential doctors in the 1930s and 1940s and that the reorientation of medical training was one of their priorities. Oxford proved to be the epicentre for the shockwaves created by the campaign and Lord Nuffield, no social medicine enthusiast himself, provided the financial support through the setting up of the Nuffield Provincial Hospitals Trust and the decisions taken by its Medical Advisory Committee.

Farquhar Buzzard was crucial to the campaign, although he seems an unlikely advocate. Translated from consultant neurological practice at St Thomas's to the Regius' Chair in Oxford in 1929, he was one of the Establishment's own. However, when in place in Oxford he exerted effective pressure for the establishment of a clinical Medical School, based on the Radcliffe Infirmary, the necessary finance to establish the four Professorships coming from Lord Nuffield.[13]

The agreement to proceed with the Oxford Medical School was finalized in the summer of 1936, the year that the BMA held its Annual Meeting in Oxford, and during which Nuffield was created an Honorary Member. It was also the year Buzzard was BMA President, giving a presidential address entitled 'And the Future.' This address, making the case for the kind of medical school which Nuffield was to bankroll, looked at the future of scientific, research-based medicine. It also spelt out a new programme for the role of hospitals and the preservation of health.

> The saving of life has become the job of institutional team-work. The saving of health and the prevention of illness, in the long run of far greater interest to the welfare of the community, must be initiated by the general practitioner in the home. I envisage great modification of both medical practice and medical education.[14]

Buzzard went no further than this in 1936, and the Oxford Medical School was planned as a training ground for research scientists, not general practitioners, but the connection between practice and education is explicit: doctors needed a new direction, and would have to be trained to be able to follow it.

At this stage another, quite different, kind of consideration was coming to bear on medical planning. In 1935 the Government had begun to prepare for a possible future European war, a war in which air power made large-scale civilian casualties a certainty. Air-raid planning was under way,[15] and naturally all the large cities were scrutinized, with London the focus of particular attention. Not only was it by far the largest centre of population but contained an exceptional concentration of doctors and many of the great teaching hospitals. It was imperative as a matter of planning to envisage the dispersal of the population (lay and professional), and the destruction, at an early stage, of the capital's medical infrastructure. At the same time issues of public health suddenly became important. Would there be epidemics in the air-raid shelters? What would be the effect of dispersing deprived city children to the countryside? Was the male population fit enough to fight? How much food was necessary to sustain the population? Ministry planners found that, in the same way as it was possible to order mass movements of the population, it became thinkable to direct a national strategy for the distribution and work of doctors. This strategy was embodied in planning for the Emergency Medical Service (EMS). The medical establishment, concentrated in hospitals liable to be obliterated, decided wisely that, although they were very much opposed to political direction of doctors, resistance to the scheme would be futile, while co-operation would allow them to remain in control of the service. From the EMS much experience of medical planning and much new thinking developed which played its part in the eventual shape of the NHS.

William Wilson Jameson was at this time Professor of Public Health and Dean at the London School of Hygiene and Tropical Medicine (LSHTM), and was very much concerned by these issues. He had long experience as a Medical Officer of Health in London, and was convinced of the need for a social approach to medical care and health planning. Through his position at LSHTM he had become adviser to Malcolm MacDonald, Minister of State at the Colonial Office. Early in the war MacDonald was moved to become Minister of Health, and he wanted Jameson as his Chief Medical Officer. Both Buzzard and Newman were involved in persuading Jameson that he should accept the offer,[16] and Jameson, wishing in any case to be in a position which he saw would be crucial in planning the post-war medical service, accepted. He was appointed in November 1940.

Before the war began there had been further important developments in Oxford which helped pave the way for the social medicine programme. Much was being made, in the late 1930s, of hospital co-ordination. Not only did common sense indicate the advantages of the sharing of hospital-based resources and expertise, but the Emergency Medical Service required it. Early in the air-raid planning activity it was realized that there was no inventory of the hospitals in the country, never mind of their facilities or the number of patients they could accommodate. A national survey was urgently instituted.[17]

In Oxford the strength of the argument for regional planning found very practical support: Lord Nuffield donated one million shares in Morris Motors to set up the Nuffield Provincial Hospitals Trust (NPHT), an organization dedicated to supporting hospital co-ordination in the provinces. The Medical Advisory Committee (MAC) of the NPHT, which in effect allocated the available funds and determined the direction of the enterprise, was chaired by Farquhar Buzzard and the Chairman of the whole Trust was Nuffield's Oxford banker William Goodenough, one of Nuffield's closest confidants and the future Chairman of the Committee which bears his name. Buzzard's power in this wealthy and influential Trust and the Trust's early activities are described elsewhere.[18, 19] The importance in relation to social medicine lies in those who were recruited to the Trust's Medical Advisory Committee and the use made of the Trust's financial power. Jameson was a founder member and was accompanied on the MAC by two others whom I have identified as central in the social medicine cause, John Ryle and James Spence. Both of these men had influence far beyond NPHT. Ryle, who was Regius Professor of Physic in Cambridge, was appointed, with NPHT funding and on the 'particular recommendation' of Buzzard, as the first Professor of Social Medicine in the country. He resigned from his Cambridge post to set up the Institute of Social Medicine in Oxford. Ryle was thoroughly dissatisfied with the way increasingly reductionist scientific medicine distanced doctors from patients' lives. In his book *Changing Disciplines*[20] he described his intellectual and vocational journey from teaching hospital physician to Professor of Social Medicine. He wrote passionately of experiences of the poverty and blighted lives he glimpsed as a medical student in the East End of London. Of hospital medicine he observed:

> I have watched disease in the ward being studied more thoroughly – if not always more thoughtfully – through the high power of the microscope .... The morbid 'material' of the hospital ward consists very largely of end result conditions for which, as a rule, only a limited amount of relief repays the long stay, the patient investigation and the anxious expectancy of the sick man or woman.[21]

Ryle was, perhaps, the most outspoken of those who saw social medicine as the means by which high-tech medicine, and thus clinical practice, would be rehumanized. In one memorable passage he articulated a central idea of those who wished to reform medical education:

> May the daily question on his [the practising doctor's] lips become not 'What is the treatment?' but 'What are the causes?' and 'If preventable, why not prevented?'[22]

There is much to connect and make natural allies of the supporters of social medicine and of those seeking the introduction of a national health service. Underlying both are ideas of equity and justice which extend beyond the consideration of the needs of individuals and into areas such as the interests of society and the role of planning. For example it was clear that, as medical, and in particular hospital, treatment became more sophisticated, there were serious inequalities in access to the best available care. At the same time it was theoretically and practically impossible to provide the very best types of care at every location. Thus provision of an equitable, accessible service required a national planning system as well as an explicitly hierarchical system of referrals between hospitals. These were precisely the issues which NPHT had been set up to promote, and an early preoccupation of the Trust was the making of precise plans for regional hospital co-ordination which they envisaged as extending, in time, to the whole country.

Other natural connections between social medicine and national health are to be found in their perspectives on populations and prevention. Social medicine involved planning for a health system designed to ensure the health of the people instead of concentrating exclusively on the health of individuals and, looking realistically at the possibilities of a welfare state, national health considerations suggested that not only was it intellectually attractive to prefer prevention to cure but that the costs of a national medical service would depend, above all, on the number of people requiring treatment for established disease.

Beveridge had this point very clearly in mind. He noted that comprehensive health and rehabilitation services were necessary for satisfactory social security, adding:

> It is a logical corollary to receipt of high benefits in disability that the individual should recognise the duty to be well and to co-operate in all steps which may lead to diagnosis of disease in early stages when it can be prevented.[23]

On the financial consequences he wrote:

> The primary interest of the Ministry of Social Security is in finding a health service which will diminish disease by prevention and cure and will ensure the careful certification needed to control payment of benefit at the rates proposed in this report.[24]

Thus by 1941 many of the conditions required to move forward proposals for both national health and social medicine were in place: the NPHT was established with a strong input from social medicine supporters. The Beveridge Committee was meeting and individuals such as Jameson, Buzzard and Dawson occupied positions of influence firmly within the mainstream of medical politics. Let us consider how these potential changes became linked to proposals for change in medical education.

The Re-evaluation of Medical Training

The philosophy of social medicine required a re-evaluation not only of the purposes of medical care but of the ways in which doctors, particularly GPs, worked. Social medicine proponents looked to a reversal of the trends which emphasized hospital-based expertise and minimized the contribution of GPs. This vision of a new role for general practitioners was more than theory. For example, the Yorkshire practitioner, William Pickles, was already working in a way which combined an acute interest in his rural community with meticulous observation and careful analysis. Pickles' seminal work *Epidemiology in a Country Practice* [25] was published in 1939 and he was invited to join NPHT in 1940, where he was admired by, and became friends with, both Ryle and Spence, who viewed him as an ideal of the practitioner of the future.[26] Any national medical system which aimed to prevent ill-health required practitioners in close contact with the people whose present and future health it was their purpose to safeguard. While necessary, this was not sufficient: prevention required doctors who were aware of predisposing risks, trained to spot illness at its very earliest stages and prepared to accept responsibility for the health of communities rather than only for individuals who were 'their' patients. This had been foreshadowed by Buzzard in 1936 and was an explicit preoccupation of Ryle.

The fact that social medicine was promoted by such powerful individuals may help to explain why, in this debate, the traditional supporters of preventive medicine, the Medical Officers of Health, appear to have been neglected. Valuable as their efforts were on behalf of the local authorities, they had specific, defined responsibilities. The new momentum required that the preventive potential in every consultation be recognized and exploited. For this to be successful all doctors and every patient would need to be involved and this neatly tied together the concepts of a universal service, effective prevention and medical education. Now that these issues were being pursued at the highest level there was a realistic chance of implementation, but the changes would only be effective if all medical practitioners were trained to play their part, not solely the Medical Officers of Health.

Doctors' training in the late 1930s paid scant attention to these matters and thus change in medical education was an essential part of furthering the ideals of social medicine. Medical education has featured little in the debates about the initiation of the NHS, and yet it might have seemed natural that there would be a close connection between a radical change in the service and an equivalent change in how medical students were prepared for their life work. The fact that this was not appreciated within medical schools and that, in the end, medical education proceeded precisely as before is strong evidence that, at least within teaching hospitals, the new service was regarded as little more than a matter of organization. Having succeeded in their effort to obtain exemption from some of the controls imposed by the NHS Act, the teaching hospital specialists could afford to assume that life, for them, would continue much as before.[27]

However, a very substantial attempt was made to radically alter medical education, to reorientate it towards a national preventive service, and place social medicine at the centre of medical training. The NPHT had been promoting plans to regionalize hospitals since the beginning of 1940. This meant making explicit links between hospitals which were close together, creating a hierarchy of expertise and an acknowledged route for referral of patients. The 'hospital centre' in each putative region was usually a teaching hospital.[28] So successful was the Trust at disseminating its ideas that serious concern developed among other interested parties. At this stage Government was uncommitted to any particular plan for post-war national health, and the local authorities, a powerful political force, were naturally alarmed at plans which took no account of traditional geographical boundaries or financial responsibilities.[29] As a result the Minister of Health made a statement in the House of Commons in October 1941[30] which committed the Government to a national hospital service after the war, but sat on the fence so far as its organization was concerned.

At the same time the setting up of an Interdepartmental Committee to consider medical education was announced. The significance of this lay in the timing of the announcement and the composition of the committee. There is no indication in the Minister's speech that the Government had any specific objective so far as education was concerned, except that the position of the teaching hospitals within a national health service had been recognized as a difficult and important issue. However, for social medicine protagonists within NPHT the announcement offered an exceptional opportunity. The Government's October 1941 announcement put an end to Nuffield regionalization plans. NPHT felt obliged to comply with a specific government request in this regard.[31] This required recompense and the Ministry was, perhaps, able to make the request because Jameson had a foot in both camps. He had experience as the Dean of a medical school and was well aware of the significance of medical education in future planning[32] and through him the interests of the Ministry, of the Nuffield Trusts and of social medicine were brought together in the Interdepartmental Committee.

NPHT was offered the chance to undertake a further national survey of hospitals and a heavy involvement in the Interdepartmental Committee on medical education. Jameson himself was set the task of constituting the committee[33] and brought in as Chairman William Goodenough, Chairman of NPHT and close Oxford associate of Buzzard and Lord Nuffield. In this way NPHT was given compensation in work of national importance and in the direction of the Interdepartmental Committee (from now on called the Goodenough Committee).

Before describing the way that social medicine ideas were incorporated in the Goodenough Report it is time to discuss two of the other central figures identified earlier: James Spence and Janet Vaughan. Both were younger Fellows of the Royal College of Physicians (RCP) and both were interested in social medicine. Spence's reputation had been made with a study of poverty and ill-health in Newcastle in the early 1930s and he was an early recruit to the MAC of NPHT. Among the indications that, by 1942, the debate surrounding social medicine had become both intense and important is that even the RCP felt obliged to take action. Janet Vaughan raised the issue in Comitia[34] and the result was the setting up of a social medicine committee by the RCP, chaired by Spence and with Vaughan as a member, which reported in October 1943.[35]

This was an interim report rapidly produced, focusing on social medicine in medical education and emphasizing the importance of social medicine to the training of doctors. The report itself formed part of the evidence of the RCP to Goodenough. Meanwhile Janet Vaughan herself had been selected as a member of the main Goodenough Committee.

Thus Beveridge, Goodenough and the RCP Committee on Social Medicine were all meeting at the same time and considering different but related aspects of the medical service, medical education and social medicine. In the middle of these deliberations Jameson made a crucial statement on behalf of social medicine, delivered as it was to the RCP in the form of one of the annual Harveian Orations.[36] This lecture was entitled 'War and the advancement of social medicine' and it was a powerful plea that the ideals of social medicine, having been given impetus by the widespread desire for change and the determination to see change implemented which arose from wartime conditions and perspectives, should be seen as an essential part of planning for the future of national health. Further, Jameson envisaged that social health would be not merely a recipient of the benefits of change, but an active agency, predicting that social medicine would be an integral part of 'some extensive programme of social reform ... introduced as an immediate post-war measure.'

At almost the same time Buzzard and Ryle were writing in the *Lancet* and *BMJ* of the need for change. Buzzard,[37] in a paper entitled 'Reconstruction in the Practice of Medicine,' identified 'three basic defects' in medical practice. These were:

1. The failure of instruction of students who were going to become general practitioners.
2. The lack of time for doctors to spend on the early detection of illness and for health promotion and disease prevention.
3. The neglect of social medicine.

Buzzard ended his paper:

> One final word. The changes in the organisation of the profession which are here suggested, must be based on changes in the education of medical students and on the intensified study of the social factors underlying the health of the nation. Prevention is better than cure.

Ryle, writing on 'Social Medicine, its Meaning and Scope,'[38] wrote:

> The practitioners of social medicine will, it need hardly be said, eventually include the whole of the practising part of the profession as well as the officers of the environmental services. There is no sharp division between individual and social medicine. Health education and periodic health examination will some day supplement the remedial activities of the general practitioner.

By late 1943, Beveridge having reported in favour of a national medical service as one of the bases for comprehensive social welfare, the RCP Social Medicine Committee having given strong support for social medicine as an essential component in the medical curriculum and the Goodenough Committee being well advanced in its taking of evidence, social medicine had been accepted as part of the mainstream of progressive thought in medical planning. Further, there is no doubting the social medicine input into the important committees: Jameson was Chief Medical Officer at the Ministry and an active member of Goodenough. Ryle was about to transfer to his new Chair in Oxford and was writing powerfully. He, Jameson, Buzzard and Spence were all heavily involved with the Nuffield Trusts. Spence chaired and Vaughan sat on the RCP Committee and Vaughan had been selected by Jameson for the Goodenough Committee.

Medical Education Reform

What of the claim which I have made that an explicit objective of the social medicine proponents was to reform medical education so as to produce doctors, and especially general practitioners, prepared for a different kind of medical practice in the National Health Service? The first evidence derives simply from an analysis of the situation. The doctors promoting social medicine were thoughtful, thorough and had a clear end in view, the transformation of social medicine ideals into the everyday practice of medicine. As such they were more aware than anyone of the deficiencies of current education, even for the old service, never mind the new.

Their new service deserved and required doctors who, even when dealing with individual patients in their care, were trained to offer advice about health preservation and to be alert to the very earliest manifestations of ill-health. The social medicine perspective emphasized, as did the concept of the NHS and the regionalization plans of NPHT, care offered to whole communities, not simply to patients on a doctor's panel or able to pay his fees. Any thoughtful individual wishing to promote social medicine would have been aware of the yawning gap between theory and practice and alert to the special place that education and training occupied in the preparation for change. Such thinking was not confined even to the active proponents of social medicine. The General Medical Council (GMC), the body with the statutory control of standards of medical education, submitted evidence to Goodenough[39] and it explicitly recognized the change of the whole emphasis of medical practice entailed by a truly socialized medical service.

In paragraph 54 of their evidence the GMC, referring to the overall aim of medical education, proposed that 'the aim is to produce a body of medical men capable of maximum service to the community.' In paragraph 56, in a specific reference to the medical curriculum, they placed promotion of health and prevention of illness on an equal footing with the treatment of disease as subjects to engage the students' attention. Such evidence of the willingness to consider change extending to the very top of the medical establishment confirms, if confirmation were needed, the great seriousness being attached to social medicine in these middle war years.

None of the exhortations for change emanating from individuals and committees makes sense unless they were intended to be translated from theory to practice and unless this practice were to be within the context of a radically reorganized medical service.

Apart from evidence derived from what individuals must have thought, what explicit written evidence is there that the educational changes were linked directly to preparation of doctors for the National

Health Service, indeed formed part of the strategy for carrying the behind-the-scenes argument for the existence of such a service?

Beveridge had laid the foundation-stone when he stated his certainty that an effective national medical service was an essential condition for making social insurance viable as a whole. The Goodenough Committee received evidence from all the interested parties and from individuals formally and informally. I have already given brief attention to the GMC's evidence. The RCP Social Medicine Committee was absolutely clear about the need for social medicine to be a compulsory undergraduate subject and why it should have a prominent place in the curriculum. The Goodenough Committee itself crystallized all this in the early paragraphs of its report: in paragraph 18, under the heading 'The dependence of a national health service on medical education' appear the words:

> Properly planned and carefully conducted medical education is *the* [their italics] essential foundation of a comprehensive medical service.

In paragraph 20, under the heading 'The effect of making the promotion of health a principal objective of the health service and of medical education,' it states:

> For some years there has been growing acceptance of the view that one of the principal aims of national policy should be to secure for everyone the highest possible standard of physical and mental health .... By becoming advisers on health both to individuals and to the community, medical practitioners will have to bear much of the responsibility for ensuring this result and by means of undergraduate and postgraduate training, must be provided with the knowledge and guidance necessary to enable them to carry out this important work. The present system of medical education is seriously deficient in this respect .... A radical reorientation of medical education and practice is essential.

The report follows this with a quotation from Lord Dawson supporting this position.[40] Later in the report, in the chapter on social medicine,[41] the point is re-emphasized:

> If students are to be fitted to become health advisers and members of a new comprehensive health service, the ideas of social medicine must permeate the whole of medical education.

It is hard to see how, following Beveridge and with the support of the RCP and the GMC, the explicit connection between the new education, the new practitioner and the new service could have been more forcibly expressed.

This being the case, how was it that the requisite radical reorientation failed to come about?

The Situation after 1945 and the Role of the GMC

The end of the war and the Labour General Election victory in 1945 changed everything. Suddenly, what had appeared, at least on the surface, to be a consensus about the need for change in medical services, became a bitter debate. The sectional interests which had been subdued during the war years recognized the threats to their individual positions. This threat was infinitely worse in the context of the Labour victory which swept Churchill and his all-party government from power. It became clear that Labour would give support to nationalization of the hospitals and the universal right to care free at the point of delivery, and that the very existence of private medical care was threatened. To doctors, whether specialists or general practitioners, ruin seemed to stare them in the face. While it had been easy enough to agree with reform in general, the details of the new service became the subject of minute scrutiny and bitter wrangling. In this context, two things happened which were fatal to the proposed reform of medical education.

The first was that the whole debate about the health service altered so that pay, conditions, compulsion and choice became the focus. Suddenly, the issues of medical education became peripheral rather than central. After all, why talk about the minutiae of training for a socialized medical service when disagreement raged about the very existence of the service?

Secondly, the teaching hospital staff had very strong reasons to object to the idea that any significant change to education was required. If the hospitals were to be nationalized it was vital that a special position be recognized for the teaching hospitals and it would hardly be politic to point out the need for radical reorganization. The teaching hospitals, particularly in London, needed financial support but were loath to concede anything else. Politically, avoiding damaging conflict with the leaders of the hospitals whose names were recognized across the country was important and the Minister of Health, Aneurin Bevan and Lord Moran, President of the RCP and chief spokesman for London consultants and the teaching hospitals, had more on their minds than the cause of social medicine.[42]

If the teaching hospitals wanted to suggest that there wasn't so much wrong with the old methods and, thus, that reform was unnecessary, the Goodenough proposals contained other serious threats to their modus operandi. Goodenough wanted teaching to be in university hands. Ever since the Flexner[43] and Haldane[44] Reports a case had been made that teaching should be administered and delivered by full-time academics and that the attention to teaching by honorary consultants whose primary interest was private practice represented a definite second best. Even by the end of the war there were few well-established professorial units within the London hospitals and they were certainly not accepted as having primacy so far as policy or teaching were concerned.[45]

Goodenough stood out for teaching departments headed by professors who would act as clinical heads and directors. The position of clinical professors as full-time university employees disbarred them from receiving additional payment for private practice and this point was, in fact, one of the reasons for preferring academic direction. It also cut the other way: those devoted to private practice could not hope or expect to be appointed to academic positions. Even before the First World War Haldane's committee reckoned, with justice, that a full-time academic salary would liberate teachers from the burdens of private practice and allow them to concentrate on their primary role, education: it is thus easy to see how, once the new health service discussion moved from generalized pronouncements to detailed planning, opinion within the teaching hospitals hardened against Goodenough. In understanding the way in which the Goodenough proposals were shelved it is essential to remember that the GMC was the body with statutory power over medical education. At the end of the war the GMC held this power by virtue of the Medical Act 1886, which gave power to inspect and approve the standard of medical schools' final examinations, but not their courses. While the GMC might make recommendations it was schools which delivered the education and answered only to themselves so far as its quality was concerned. Of the members of the GMC in 1945 two-thirds held their place as the representative of the very universities and schools whose education was deemed to be unsuitable. Whatever fine words appeared in reports and although the members of the Goodenough Committee had satisfied themselves that the hospitals were on their side, the reality was that the teaching hospital staffs, as a group and individually, could decide whether change would or would not occur.

And yet it was not possible simply to deny Goodenough. There were powerful voices for change and the new Government, while not having education as a particular priority, wished to see the new NHS firmly established. Much of Jameson's thinking was in tune with Nye Bevan's programme and Bevan credited Jameson in large measure with the successful introduction of the service.[46]

In the interval between the publication of Goodenough and the end of the war, the GMC had acted to begin the process of implementation. To this end four parallel committees were established to undertake a major review of the curriculum reflecting the then state of GMC thinking that promotion of health and prevention of illness must be enhanced in the curriculum.[47] The committees were charged with reviewing pre-medical, pre-clinical, clinical and social medicine and public health training. Social medicine was thus given a status equal to the whole of the rest of clinical medicine and change seemed merely a matter of time. However, while the committees talked the war ended, and with political change came the realization and realities to which I have already referred. Progress ceased, and by early in 1946 the four committees were no longer meeting. Agreement on curricular change had not been reached and a delegation, paid for by the Nuffield Provincial Hospitals Trust and the Rockefeller Foundation, was dispatched to seek guidance from American universities, some of which had sophisticated departments of public health and medical schools which were highly integrated with their parent universities.

After a prolonged delay (27 months from the establishment of the committees) draft recommendations on medical education were submitted to the Council on 25 February 1947 and adopted as the recommendations on medical education to the licensing bodies. In these recommendations it can be seen that a battle had been fought and lost. Social medicine, which underpinned both the most radical ideas about the role of a comprehensive health service and the argument for fundamental changes in education, had been almost erased from the agenda. A careful comparison of the GMC educational recommendations of 1936[48] and 1947[49] shows that, in spite of the wartime rhetoric, social medicine received, if anything, even less recognition in the curriculum after the war than before it. The NHS, through its virtual absence from the documents, was clearly not seen within the GMC to require, of itself, educational change. Not only did social medicine (scornfully dismissed as 'those aspects of medicine as a whole which are now often comprehensively described as "social medicine"') come far down the list of priorities, but the proposed method of instructing students was through local authority and social work services distanced physically, and even more importantly philosophically, from the thrust of scientific training envisaged elsewhere in the recommendations.

This blow, coupled with the medical brinkmanship and political turmoil associated with the arguments and final acceptance of the reality of the NHS, pushed social medicine off the agenda and into the backwater from which it has never emerged. This is partly due to the development of disciplines (public health, epidemiology, medical sociology) which might have been considered as falling within the remit of a broader discipline called social medicine. But why, after drawing breath and while working within a service which provided ample opportunities to continue to work with social medicine ideals, the power of the social medicine protagonists was so completely eclipsed remains a question which has not yet been fully explored. Although Ryle's Unit of Social Medicine in Oxford was followed by the establishment of others, for example under Thomas McKeown in Birmingham and F. A. E. Crew in Edinburgh, they each pursued their own agenda, losing the social medicine emphasis on education. Various possible reasons spring to mind: the defeat in the GMC and the confirmation of the teaching hospitals' autonomy may have been hard to bear; the Units may have felt a need to concentrate first on establishing the scientific claims of a social approach to medicine; the activists may merely have become more interested in other things. In my interview with Dame Janet Vaughan I asked her if she felt very disappointed with the fate of the Goodenough Report. She replied that she hadn't really thought about it: the Government had asked her to lead a research group on the effects of radioactive Strontium, and that had occupied her completely. Nevertheless, the loss of virtually the whole of the preventive medicine agenda in the early years of the NHS is hard to explain and would repay detailed study.

Perhaps the eventual outcome was foreseen by N. M. Goodman and Jerry Morris in an article written in 1940 and entitled 'The Clinical Teaching of Social Medicine.'[50]

> At the end of the war the question of whether the social services are to be sacrificed on the altar of economy may well depend on whether the medical profession regard them as something outside their province or as an essential weapon in the fight for health.

The medical establishment, embodied in the GMC, made its decision with a ruthless rejection of the social medicine argument.

Notes

1. The Interdepartmental Committee on Medical Schools (Goodenough Committee) (London: HMSO, 1944), 167. This was the committee established to review the position of medical schools and the role they would play in the proposed changes to medical services after the Second World War. It is worth noting that social medicine, in particular in its preventive aspects, had been introduced into many medical schools in the USA in the 1930s. J. G. Fitzgerald *Journal of the American Medical Association*, 110 (1938), 1321–6, reported that 18 out of a responding group of 69 medical schools had full-time university departments of preventive medicine, public health and hygiene.
2. C. Webster, *Health Services Since the War*, Vol. 1 (London: HMSO, 1988), 2–15.
3. Rudolf Klein, *The Politics of the National Health Service* (Harlow: Longman, 1983).
4. Webster, *op.cit.*, ch. 2, 16–43.
5. George Newman, *Infant Mortality: A Social Problem* (London: Methuen, 1906).
6. *Royal Commission on the Poor Law, Report* (London: HMSO, 1909, Cmnd, 4449).
7. S. Webb and B. Webb, *The State and the Doctor* (London: Longmans & Green, 1910), v.
8. Consultative Council on Medical and Allied Services, *Interim Report 1920* (*The Dawson Report*) (London: HMSO, Cmnd 693).
9. *Ibid*., para. 6.
10. Innes Pearse and G. S. Williamson, *The Case for Action* (London: Faber, 1931). The preface was written by A. D. Lindsay, Professor of Moral Philosophy at Oxford from 1924 and Vice-Chancellor 1935–8. He was well known for his progressive views and was another connection with those Oxford-based individuals whose names will recur throughout this chapter.
11. Innes Pearse and Lucy Crocker, *The Peckham Experiment* (London: Allen & Unwin, 1943).
12. Lord Dawson, House of Lords, 24 February 1943.
13. Sir Douglas Veale in 'The Nuffield Benefaction and the Oxford Medical School,' in Kenneth Dewhurst, *Oxford Medicine* (Oxford: Oxford University Press, 1970), 143–53.
14. Sir Farquhar Buzzard, 'And the future,' *British Medical Journal*, 2 (1936), 165.
15. C. L. Dunn, *History of the Second World War. The Emergency Medical*

Services, Vol. 1 (London: HMSO, 1952).

16. N. M. Goodman, *William Jameson, Architect of National Health* (London: Allen & Unwin, 1970), 81.
17. C. L. Dunn, *op.cit.*, 14.
18. Nuffield Provincial Hospitals Trust, *A Report on the Purposes and Activities of the Trust 1939–1948* (Oxford: Oxford University Press, 1949).
19. N. T. A. Oswald, 'A Social Health Service Without Doctors,' *Social History of Medicine*, 4 (1991), 295-315; 300.
20. J. A. Ryle, *Changing Disciplines* (Oxford: Oxford University Press – 1948), ch. 3.
21. *Ibid.*, 19–20.
22. *Ibid.*, 23.
23. *Social Insurance and Allied Services* (*Beveridge Report*) (London: HMSO, 1942, Cmnd 6404), para. 426.
24. *Ibid.*, para. 437.
25. William Pickles, *Epidemiology in a Country Practice* (Bristol: Wright, 1939).
26. John Pemberton, *Will Pickles of Wensleydale* (London: Bles, 1970), 123–4.
27. The teaching hospitals were considered separately from all other hospitals in the nationalization/regionalization plans which accompanied the introduction of the NHS. Webster, *op.cit.* (ref. 2), 270.
28. NPHT was concerned exclusively with the provinces and could thus afford to ignore the difficult problem of what 'regionalization' might mean within the metropolis.
29. Geoffrey Rivett, *The Development of the London Hospital System 1823–1982* (London: King Edward's Hospital Fund for London, 1986), ch. 10.
30. Government statement on post-war hospital policy (Hansard 1940–1, Vol. 374, column 1116–18).
31. Nuffield Trust, *op.cit.* (ref. 18), 13.
32. He had formed a personal 'think tank' called the 'Gasbag Committee' to consider such issues before the war, and while still at the London School of Hygiene.
33. Goodman, *op.cit.* (ref. 16), 140.
34. According to her account she was the first woman ever to have spoken in Comitia (Dame Janet Vaughan, personal interview, Oxford, December 1987).
35. Royal College of Physicians of London, *Interim Report of the Social and Preventative Medicine Committee* (London, October 1943).

36. William Wilson Jameson, 'War and the Advancement of Social Medicine,' *Lancet*, ii, (1942), 475–80.
37. Sir E. Farquhar Buzzard, 'Reconstruction in the Practice of Medicine,' *Lancet*, i (1942), 343–7.
38. J. A. Ryle, 'Social Medicine, its Meaning and Scope,' *British Medical Journal*, ii (1943), 633–6.
39. GMC, *Minutes* (1943), 159–200.
40. Sir Bertrand Dawson, House of Lords, 24 February 1943.
41. Interdepartmental Committee, *op.cit.* (ref.1), ch. 11.
42. Moran hated both Jameson and Ryle, and was active in opposing them in the RCP (Sir George Godber, personal communication).
43. *Medical Education in the United States and Canada*, Carnegie Foundation, *Bulletin* 4 (1910) (*Flexner Report*).
44. Royal Commission on University Education in London, *Blue Books* Vol. xi (London: HMSO, 1913) (*Haldane Report*).
45. PRO MH71/75, 29 June 1943. This issue was specifically addressed by the Dean of St Thomas's, Professor McSwiney, who, in evidence to Goodenough, indicated his staff's acceptance of reform in general but explicitly rejected primacy for academic departments.
46. Goodman, *op.cit.* (ref.16), 120–1.
47. General Medical Council, *Minutes* (1944), 73.
48. General Medical Council, 'Resolutions in Regard to Professional Education', *Minutes* (1936), Appendix 9.
49. General Medical Council, 'Recommendations as to Medical Education', *Minutes* (1947), Appendix 3.
50. N. M. Goodman and Jerry Morris, 'The Clinical Teaching of Social Medicine,' *Proceedings of the Royal Society of Medicine*, 33 (1940), 751–6.

3

Making Medicine Social: The Case of the Two Dogs with Bent Legs

Ann Oakley

This chapter discusses the evolution of social medicine in Britain from a particular biographical perspective: that of Richard Titmuss, who played a key role in some of the early social medicine work, publishing a series of joint papers with Jerry Morris on social inequalities in health. Titmuss was Deputy Director of the Medical Research Council's first institutional foray into the business of social medicine – the Social Medicine Research Unit – for two years before moving on to his longer and better-known sojourn as Professor in the Department of Social Administration at the London School of Economics (LSE). Using the context of the Titmuss Papers,[1] this chapter attempts to provide some kind of sociological answer to the questions: what was social medicine, where did it come from, and what happened to it?

Of Mice and Dogs

The 'case of the two dogs with bent legs' is a phrase taken from Chapter 1 of J. B. S. Haldane's *Heredity and Politics,* published in 1938. The book addresses the relevance to contemporary social and political questions of recently acquired knowledge about human biology. This, of course, was in a context in which biological arguments were currently being used to justify social policies of quite drastic kinds, including the oppression of Jews in Nazi Germany and the sterilization in both right- and left-wing countries of individuals assessed as 'mentally defective.' Haldane points out that most such biological arguments refer for their rationale to genetics. The history of genetics itself shows an overwhelming focus on the explanation of differences, rather than resemblances. Because of this, 'It is possible,' says Haldane, 'to give a reasonable answer to the question, "Why is this mouse black while this other mouse is white?" but at present it is not possible to give at all an adequate answer to the question, "Why are they both mice? Why does a pair of mice produce another mouse and not a rat or a motor-bicycle?"' One problem about genetic arguments is their weakness on the topic of causation. 'Let us suppose,' continues Haldane, 'that we have before us two dogs, both with legs somewhat bent. It may be that one of these dogs has bent legs because as a puppy it received a diet containing inadequate quantities of anti-rachitic vitamin, while the other dog has bent legs because its father was a dachshund. In the first case we say that the difference between this dog and a straight-legged dog is due to nurture. In the second case we say that it is due to nature. It is possible by experimental methods with animals and plants to separate these two causes of variation, but ... in the majority of cases both of the causes are operative .... In man, where experiment is impossible, we shall find it very much harder to determine the origin of the differences that undoubtedly exist' (Haldane, 1938: 24–5).

Haldane's statement of the role of the biological and the social in determining human physique sums up a crucial theme leading to the development of social medicine: the need which was felt in certain academic, political and scientific quarters at the time, to take issue with current influential biological views of health. This process of countering biological determinist claims provided a profound impetus to socialize medicine in two distinct though overlapping senses – firstly, *theories* underlying medicine about health and disease were driven to expand and take in the realm of the social, and, secondly, awareness of the role of the social in shaping health and disease outcomes highlighted the desirability of socializing medical *practice,* that is, of making medical services equally available to all citizens in the form of a state-funded health service. The rest of this chapter illustrates and develops these points by looking in more detail at the development of Titmuss's own work within the context of contemporary understandings and practices relating to health. I shall argue that the emergence of the concept of social class as a variable consistently associated with health outcomes was crucial to the wider conceptualization of social medicine as a legitimate scientific area of study.

Grading Eggs and Classing Men

For most of the first half of the twentieth century, public discourses about health in the UK and many other countries were dominated by the terminology of eugenics. The quality of the population was the major public health concern. The story of how the physical standard of recruits for military service provided a measure of population quality from the Boer War onwards is a familiar one (see Teitelbaum and Winter, 1985), and it is repeated in the history of the Second World War, too.

Francis Galton, a cousin of Charles Darwin, defined eugenics in a lecture to the Sociological Society in 1904 as 'the science which deals with all influences that improve the inborn qualities of a race; also with those that develop them to the utmost advantage' (Galton, 1909). The Eugenic Education Society, as it was originally called, was founded in 1907. Included in its aims were promoting eugenist ideals in parenthood, and dissemination in schools and elsewhere of information about the laws of heredity as applied to racial improvement. There are many accounts of the rise, composition and influence of the eugenics movement (see e.g. Jones, 1986; Mackenzie, 1976; Searle, 1979), and I do not intend to duplicate these here, except to note several key characteristics of the movement which were germaine to the development of social medicine. The first is that the eugenics movement was remarkably widespread in its coverage of key figures in the British social, political and health landscape. For example, it included Keynes, Beveridge, Eleanor Rathbone, Marie Stopes, Julian Huxley, Cyril Burt, the Webbs, Harold Laski, Eva Hubback, Havelock Ellis, J. W. B. Douglas, and Eysenck among its members. Almost everybody who was somebody belonged. A second important point is that the movement embraced people with a very wide range of social backgrounds and political interests. While aristocratic names were associated with it, so were socially mobile industrialists (see Jones, 1986) and well-known charitable families such as the Cadburys and the Rowntrees. Indeed, there was a strong sense in which alliance with the eugenics movement marked a commitment to social reform. The third point is that the eugenics movement in the UK found itself in particular difficulty in the late 1930s and 1940s for obvious reasons to do both with events in Germany and with increasingly worsening domestic social conditions associated with unemployment (which put a considerable strain on traditional eugenic theories of joblessness being a form of congenital abnormality). While individual Eugenics Society members' political viewpoints might not have been all that far removed from some of the policies of Nazism, there were many others within the movement who were keen to disassociate British eugenics from these highly distasteful developments.

In 1937, Richard Titmuss was working as an Inspector for a large insurance company in London, but he had for some years been pursuing a complementary evening and weekend career as a statistician. His first publications on vital statistics were in the insurance press. For example, in an article entitled 'The Birth Rate and Insurance,' published in the *Post Magazine and Insurance Monitor* in 1936, he argued that those working in the fire and accident insurance industry needed to be aware that the future of the business was in jeopardy, since projections of population needs forecast a progressively ageing population; not enough babies were being born to provide the insurance industry with future work. Titmuss himself was clearly more interested in the substantive issue here than in what might happen to insurance. In the mid-1930s he met his future wife, Kathleen Miller, whose social work among London's unemployed helped to focus his work more sharply on social issues. Titmuss's first – unpublished – book, called *Crime and Tragedy*, was a passionate, though rather badly written, attack on the machinations of governments and political leaders, particularly in Britain, against the interests of world peace. The book was written under the pseudonym of 'Richard Caston,' for fear that the insurance company that employed him would find out what he was up to. He sent the manuscript to the *News Chronicle* who turned it down, and then to Sylvia Pankhurst for possible serialization in her journal *New Times and Ethiopia News*. She did offer to publish part of it, but as he asked for a fee of £2 and she refused to pay anything, it never saw the light of day (Titmuss Papers (TP), Pankhurst to RMT, 13.11.37).

The year Sylvia Pankhurst turned down *Crime and Tragedy*, Titmuss went to a Eugenics Society lecture on population trends given by the social statistician R. Kuczynski. This so impressed him that he immediately asked to join the Society. He became a member in 1937, and a Fellow and member of Council in 1939; during the war he served on the Emergency Committee and was acting editor for several issues of the *Eugenics Review*. The Society helped to fund the publication of his second book, and also several other initiatives in which he was involved. He resigned from the Society because of overwork 17 days before his death in 1973.

In 1938, Titmuss's first book on social statistics was published. *Poverty and Population* was subtitled 'A Factual Study of Contemporary Social Waste.' The book is concerned with the numerical importance and incidence of preventable and premature death associated with poor diet and other unhealthy environmental factors, and was written primarily to argue the case for a link between poverty and mortality. (It also, incidentally, pursued Titmuss's interest in the health of army recruits, analysing this by region, and showing that rejection rates in the North were 50–80% higher than in the Home Counties (Titmuss, 1938: 66). Titmuss later became adviser on German statistics to the Ministry of Economic Warfare.) The main statistics of social difference drawn on in *Poverty and Population* were regional ones, though Titmuss also made some use of unemployment figures, and data on housing density. After looking at a number of childhood and adult mortality rates, Titmuss concluded that some 50,000 men, women and children were dying every year of preventable deaths, that is deaths primarily due to environmental, and therefore correctable, causes.

Poverty and Population carried a preface by Lord Horder – physician to the Royal family and president of the Eugenics Society from 1935. Titmuss solicited the writing of this preface, which amounted to Eugenics Society sponsorship of the book, through his connection with the Society. The book received much press attention under headings such as 'Two Nations. The North and the South' (*Yorkshire Observer*, 21.11.39), 'Social Waste – State Must Intervene' (*Chester Chronicle*, 12.11.38), '50,000 Condemned to Die of Poverty' (*Daily Herald*, 28.10.38), and 'Britain's Peril of Extinction – Serious Threats to our Racial Stock' (*Sheffield Telegraph*, 3.11.38).

By this time, Titmuss was heavily involved in many Eugenics Society activities. These included negotiations with Sir Sylvanus Vivian, the Registrar-General, for improving routine official statistics, on behalf of the Population Investigation Committee (PIC) which had been set up by the Society and was then headed by Carr-Saunders, Chair of the Leverhulme Committee who funded some of Titmuss's work, and Director of the LSE and Titmuss's sponsor there. The PIC and Titmuss wanted more routine recording of information, such as maternal age on birth registration forms and marital status on (men's) death certificates. As Titmuss put it – in the kind of purple prose of which he was fond at the time (and out of which his wife tried to educate him) – 'We can grade our eggs, count our cows, pigs and potatoes, know the birthdays of filmstars and carefully preserve stags and foxes for socially canonised carnage but we cannot tell the average age of our mothers when they produce' (TP, RMT, unpublished paper, probably 1936).

Critical to Titmuss's relationship with the Eugenics Society was the development of his association with Maurice Newfield, editor of the *Eugenics Review* from 1933 on. Newfield's appointment had itself been a challenging one for the Society, as he was strongly associated with the birth control movement and regarded for this reason as a potentially controversial figure. In December 1939, Newfield described in a letter to Titmuss a conversation he had had recently with Lord Horder in which they had both decided that 'during the war our primary functions would be to restate eugenic principles in contemporary terms (which would mean emphasising far more than we did in the past the eugenic significance of nutritional and other environmental factors), to stress the differences between eugenics and Nazi eugenics, 'butter *not* guns; genes *not* blood; the health of the individual *not* the right of the State...' (TP, Maurice Newfield to RMT, 6.10.39). Newfield went on to ask Titmuss whether he would make available to him 'anything whatever in the form of articles or annotations or other items, that may help to further our present purposes.' François Lafitte, secretary of the Population Investigation Committee, later leader writer on *The Times* and Professor at Birmingham, and David Glass, of LSE fame, had already promised such help. Newfield's view was that he had here the 'nucleus of a team' that could do much 'to liberalize eugenic thought and policies in the difficult days ahead.'

Titmuss replied the next day in positive terms, noting that he had already taken a step in the right direction by inviting Margery Spring Rice to address the Society on the findings of her survey of the health of working-class wives (TP, RMT to Maurice Newfield, 7.12.39). His letter to her recommended a 'frank and hard-hitting address on the abject monotony and drabness of the life of the average mother,' and said this should do the Fellows and Members of the Society a lot of good, as most of them had no conception of what living in poverty meant (TP, RMT to Margery Spring Rice, 20.12.39). In Titmuss's subsequent correspondence with Newfield there is much discussion of the material with which they both had to work in reshaping the philosophy and practice of eugenics. Newfield referred to 'medievally minded ladies and gentlemen' who were 'reactionary, class conscious and concerned with eugenics mainly as a doctrine that justifies its dislike of the lower orders and more particularly of the social services from which these would benefit' (TP, Maurice Newfield to RMT, 13.12.39). Titmuss complained about the petty behaviour of Council members, who haggled over money and yet treated themselves to 'marvellous' lunches of 'chicken, tongue, salad, soup, drinks, coffee, etc., and cigarettes provided free which must ... cost £25 a year' (TP, RMT to KCT, 28.11.39). Newfield pleaded with Titmuss not to regard the reactionary behaviour of Council members as evidence that the Society was beyond salvation. The thing was just to go ahead and do and say what was needed: 'If you want to put over any revolutionary idea you please, all you have to do is to call it eugenics...' (TP, Maurice Newfield to RMT, 13.12.39).

In 1942 Titmuss's published work began to focus more specifically on birth, birth rates and infant mortality. *Parents Revolt*, a book published jointly with Kathleen Titmuss, developed the argument about differential fertility along lines that would not have been unrecognizable to some of the medievally minded eugenists: the Titmusses welcomed the decrease in the class differential in fertility on the grounds that this would reduce the dysgenic effect of the poor reproducing more than the rich (Titmuss and Titmuss, 1942). *Birth, Poverty and Wealth*, published the following year (Titmuss, 1943), was described by Titmuss overtly as a 'study of inequality'; it was originally to be called *Poor Children Die* (TP, KCT to Myant, 26.2.42). The book got Titmuss into considerable trouble with the Eugenics Society, as they had given him a subsidy for the work, but had evidently not quite known what they were buying. When the manuscript was finished, members of the Council took it home with them, and the result was eight pages of criticism condemning the book as 'a political diatribe' (TP, RMT to J. N. Morris, 20.6.42). Carr-Saunders, in particular, complained that Titmuss's analysis played down the real importance of hereditary factors.

In *Birth, Poverty and Wealth*, Titmuss moved from examining regional influences on life chances to looking at occupational ones. Just as *Poverty and Population* had shown that biological determinist arguments about health could not explain regional differences in life chances, so *Birth, Poverty and Wealth* demonstrated the inability of such theories to explain social class differences. Titmuss's method was to take the Registrar-General's occupationally based social classes and rework the figures, omitting those occupations in which the mix of skill level and/or economic rewards were in his view likely to have confused the picture. The results showed a threefold increase in mortality from the highest to the lowest classes in two time periods, 1911 and 1930–2. Comparing the two time periods, there was no overall decrease in the social class gradient. But Titmuss went on to unpack the child mortality rates and to demonstrate a crucial difference between early and late infant mortality. While there had been a general decrease in the excess Class V mortality in the first month of life since 1911, there had been a 200% increase in the 6–12-month age group. This, he argued, disproved eugenist claims about biological determinants of health, as the biological argument could not explain why infant mortality appeared to be especially sensitive to the social conditions obtaining in later infancy.

To medical sociologists and epidemiologists in the 1990s, this analysis of mortality by social class seems an absolutely unremarkable exercise, and, indeed, one that does not explain very much. Social class is itself the phenomenon to be explained; occupationally based class groupings are only crude indicators of material conditions, they do not adequately represent the social positions of women, and those who grapple with social class statistics have to deal with the complex and complicating issues of the way in which individuals and groups may move both downwards and upwards for reasons which are themselves related to inequalities in health status (see Illsley, 1980). However, it is very important to realize that the technique Titmuss used, of calculating the 'excess' mortality of one occupational grouping over that of another, had not been tried before in analysing British health statistics, although it had been established via the work of Grotjahn and others in German social medicine for some time (Grotjahn, 1923). Use of the method provided crucial comparative evidence of the relationship between social circumstances and life chances. In the face of this, it became simply much more difficult to argue that people who died early or became ill did so because of the constitutional qualities with which they had been born. The careful statistical accounting engaged in by Titmuss did succeed in pushing eugenist thought further away from the biological model of health towards one that paid real attention to the significance of social factors. Crucial to this shift was the reframing of the concept of 'class' itself, from having a primarily biological, to having instead a social, referent. This process of redefinition and statistical demonstration was, significantly, one of mutual benefit for both Titmuss and the Eugenics Society; the Society achieved from Titmuss's work a more respectable image based on 'hard' statistics establishing a social model of health and illness, and Titmuss himself gained an entrée to circles of influence that helped him to emerge from the obscurity of the insurance world to a position of international importance in the social and health policy field (see Oakley, 1996).

From Eugenics to Social Medicine

As others have observed (see e.g. Porter and Porter, 1988), the term 'social medicine' has been interpreted in various ways; it has historical and contemporary alliances with other terms, including social hygiene, public health, preventive medicine, medical sociology, community medicine and, most recently, the sociology of health and illness. Each term sums up the fashions of its own epoch and has overlaps with others, but there are also important and fundamental differences. 'Social medicine' is not a concept that occurred in Titmuss's work for the Eugenics Society, nor did it feature in his early books. The primary drift of his work was epidemiological; 'sociographic' rather than sociological. Titmuss's primary intention was to chart the relationship between social conditions and health outcomes, including within this an expanded notion of the outcomes that were looked at, that is, to cover 'disease' as well as mortality, and notions of positive health as well as illness. This latter ambition was severely restricted by the raw statistical material on which any analysis had to draw, and remains so today. A related methodological point is that the rooting of social medicine in the instrument of the social survey was, as Armstrong (Armstrong, 1983) has demonstrated, also a means of its limitation, not essentially in its method so much as in the conception underlying and fuelling it. The survey was a means of collecting information from, and about, individuals relevant to health and needed to supplement crude mortality data in order to give a wider picture of health which included the social. Any broader conception of what surveys might do in terms of understanding the social relations of health had to wait until the later development of medical sociology in the 1970s, with its understanding of the key role of other methods of collecting health data, including, most importantly, those of in-depth so-called 'qualitative' interviewing and detailed ethnographic observation (see Stacey, 1988). Here a crucial theme concerns the efforts of social science in the earlier period to establish itself as a discipline complementary to, if not equal in importance to, that of medicine in understanding health and illness. The social survey was the means by which social scientists could obtain and analyse objective data objectively (Caradog Jones, n.d.); in this sense, it was the social equivalent of the medical examination, with its associated paraphernalia of laboratory tests and other 'objective' technologies.

Other developments in the field of social medicine were occurring at the same time as Titmuss's labours with vital statistics. It was these, and particularly his meeting and subsequent working partnership with Jerry Morris, that appear to have introduced into his work the language of social medicine. In 1941, Titmuss joined a group called the Committee for the Study of Social Medicine which met under the chairmanship of Professor A. St G. Huggett at St

Mary's Hospital (Titmuss became Vice-Chair). The term 'social medicine' was not widely used until 1942 (see Lewis, 1986), and it is about this time that Titmuss himself starts to use it. On the level of his own research studies, social medicine is part of a wide and ambitious project conceived with Morris, in which the idea of social medicine was to be taken forward through statistical and other forms of research to reshape both health policy and medical practice; the end result was to be a profound health-promoting impact on the welfare of the community at large. Titmuss and Morris's project was to involve 'two readerships, two cottages, and two season tickets' (TP, KCT to J. N. Morris, 5.12.42) and a book which was to be a 'masterpiece on Social Medicine' (TP, KCT to J. N. Morris, 16.11.42). Titmuss was particularly impressed by hearing John Ryle, Britain's first Professor of Social Medicine, lecture in late 1942, particularly as Ryle took the view that the whole activity of social medicine in Britain was justified by the work that Titmuss and Morris themselves were doing. The three papers they published between 1942 and 1944 were hailed by Ryle as the 'first example of a practical social medicine' (TP, KCT to K. C. Miller, 8.10.42).

The papers were concerned respectively with the epidemiology of juvenile rheumatism (Morris and Titmuss, 1942), the history of rheumatic heart disease (Morris and Titmuss, 1944a), and the epidemiology of peptic ulcer (Morris and Titmuss, 1944b). These three health conditions were picked for study because of their association with social factors. The analyses in the three papers continued the careful statistical work begun by Titmuss, but now as part of a very much broader and ambitious plan to create a comprehensive map of the ways in which different indices of social and material conditions were related to different health outcomes. Built into this was a *dynamic* view of social medicine as being about the measurement of changing health states in changing social conditions. In their rheumatic heart disease paper, for example, Morris and Titmuss plotted the relationship between rheumatic heart disease mortality as a 'social disease' against an index of social conditions based on unemployment rates over the period from 1927 to 1938; they concluded that a positive relationship existed which was strengthened when a mortality lag of three years was introduced into the analysis.

As part of their transcontinental correspondence, Titmuss and Morris drafted in 1942 a paper on the meaning of social medicine (TP, RMT to J. N. Morris, 7.12.42). This began with the words, 'Social Medicine deals with the social relations of health.' The qualification, 'A sweeping definition perhaps but not a restricting one' written by Morris, was crossed out by Titmuss. The paper went on to argue that world-wide civil war had been in part responsible for the birth of social medicine, which was therefore inevitably tied to social freedom; that is, to the reconstruction work anticipated when the war ended. In addition, social medicine was said to embrace the notion of multiple factors causing disease and disorder, rather than the earlier single factorial model, and to exemplify an emphasis on 'the study of life' rather than 'a morbid concentration on death.' In the study of life, Titmuss and Morris saw the assessment and definition of health needs as all-important. A paragraph headed 'Social Medicine at Work' read as follows:

> Because health itself has become so much a social phenomenon and because health services will increasingly be social services; because, in short, medicine is so much mixed up with society, their conjoint study emerges as a key subject. Social Medicine is medicine in the matrix of society, it studies health and the health services in the context of the society which in so great a measure conditions them. It integrates medicine with the social sciences. It is concerned with individual health but recognizes that the whole man cannot be studied except as a member of his community. The scope of Social Medicine is co-extensive with the impact of society on the health of its members.

In the second part of their draft paper, Morris and Titmuss argued the case for a health charter which would extend to health Beveridge's acceptance of the principle of 'essential needs' in relation to the social services. Such a charter would imply fundamental research into the relationship between living conditions and health, including the impact on mental health of the growing social isolation of man in his urban environment.

Titmuss and Morris's first paper on juvenile rheumatism appeared in the *Lancet* at the same time as the founding of the Oxford Institute of Social Medicine was announced. The programme of work on social medicine envisaged by Titmuss and Morris was given an institutional base with the MRC's funding of the Social Medicine Research Unit in 1948. The agenda proposed for the SMRU by Titmuss and Morris identified three underlying principles: first, the marriage of vital statistics with local social and medical enquiries; second, morbidity studies using data generated by the NHS and National Insurance Acts; third, research into 'the actual operation of social-medical services' (TP, unpublished paper, 3.1.47). This joint programme of social medicine work was brought to an unanticipated early end when Titmuss left to join LSE two years later. Although he pursued an interest in class inequalities throughout his life, after 1950 class and health was not the central research theme it had been before this.

Social Medicine or a Medicine of the Social?

What was the relationship between Titmuss's work and the wider project of which social medicine was a part? First of all, it could be argued that Titmuss's work was the key both to the development of social medicine and to what one might describe as its untimely premature death. The development of social medicine was crucially tied to three contemporary issues: the crisis in eugenic thinking about health, the move towards a state-funded health service, and the particular visionary circumstances of world-wide war: that paradox, well illustrated in Titmuss's own later social history of health policy in wartime, *Problems of Social Policy* (Titmuss, 1950), that, while war is a means of major destruction, it is also good for civilian health. One important underlying mechanism here is the effect war has of focusing the practical attention of policy-makers on the material and social basis of health – on that very environmental frame of reference that is at the heart of social medicine in its various, changing guises. But it was, as others have argued (Lewis, 1986), partly this intimate relationship between social medicine and the socio-political climate of the times that rendered it vulnerable, that militated against its survival as a strong and autonomous voice in academic and policy circles. Other reasons included disputes between key figures about what exactly social medicine was, the failure of the discipline – if discipline it was – to develop any autonomous theoretical base, and the search for academic credibility, which drove a wedge between social medicine as an academic subject, on the one hand, and public health, as that area of work concerned with the *practical* implications of the social relations of health, on the other.

The extent to which definitions of social medicine embraced political values was fiercely debated. There was a growing rift here between Titmuss and Morris on the one hand, and Ryle on the other. Ryle's version of social medicine saw it as a kind of social statistical addendum to the clinical model of health and disease. He contended that social medicine was in essence no more nor less than 'a direct development and expansion of clinical medicine' (Ryle, 1943: 4324), and argued that, although social medicine had developed at the same time as an interest in State medicine, the two had nothing essentially to do with one another. Ryle was referring here in part to a whole history of suspicion about the sociological enterprise. In greeting the birth of the Oxford Social Medicine Institute in 1942, the *British Medical Journal*, for example, referred to the founding of the Section of Medical Sociology within the British Medical Association in 1908 when the view that sociology equalled socialism had apparently carried some weight (Editorial, 1942).

Ryle, then, was a particular disappointment to social medicine, and although Alice Stewart took over the Directorship of the Oxford Unit when Ryle died in 1950, the University was sufficiently unenlightened not to make her a professor (Webster, 1986). (The differential treatment of issues to do with men and women is actually a considerable subtext in all of this.) Secondly, Titmuss himself did not invent social medicine. Rather, he seized the opportunity to relate his own work to this. There were strong ideological attractions for him in social medicine, particularly as, whatever Ryle said, social medicine *was* grounded in a political view of health. But behind Titmuss's alliance with social medicine there was also a practical motivation for someone who had left school at 15 without any formal academic qualifications and who did not want to spend the rest of his life in the insurance industry. Although Titmuss's early life was unfavourable to the growth of any kind of scientist, it is interesting to note that he himself was not averse to claiming an hereditary bent in the direction of social medicine; his mother's family were Farrs, and he claimed descent from Dr William Farr, first statistician to Britain's Registrar-General and author of *Vital Statistics,* a work which Titmuss would have been proud to have authored; before William in the family tree was also Dr Samuel Farr, who in 1780 published Hippocrates' epidemiological treatises (TP, RMT to B. Hargreaves, 2.1.38).

Thirdly, the definitional vagueness that accompanied social medicine through its brief career was reflected in Titmuss's own position, which remained ambiguous, if not ambivalent, on several key points. Some of the remarks which preface his early publications in the field and which indicate an acceptance of eugenist principles were undoubtedly put there to gain credibility and help to shift the eugenic vision away from biology and towards the social environment – it is not possible or sensible to distinguish the strength of the two motives here. But some strands of Titmuss's social medicine work did reflect a limiting concern with traditional approaches to social categorization. Included here is his work for the Eugenics Society Problem Families Committee in 1948, which focused on identifying the increasingly common phenomenon of problem families defined by 'intractable ineducability', 'infirm character,' 'fecklessness,' and 'squalor' in either the head of the household or the 'housewife' – though most commonly, the Committee decided, the housewife (Problem Families Committee, 1948).

Finally, it is, of course, inappropriate to judge the achievements of one generation by the standards of another; time moves on, and with it the possibility for enlarging and altering human understanding, and reshaping what knowledge itself may be considered to be. Some of what Titmuss and others were trying to do in developing the project of social medicine was limited by the material available. His and Morris's work on unemployment and mortality, for example, tangled with a subject that has proved notoriously difficult to analyse, even with much more sophisticated statistical evidence and techniques (Bartley, 1992). The tension between biological and social explanations which gave birth to social medicine was not new, and the distinction between nature and nurture could, and can, rarely be expressed so cleanly as in Haldane's metaphor of dogs with bent legs. It could be argued that part of the failure of social medicine to survive and transform itself into the study of the social relations of health envisaged by Titmuss and others derived precisely from its enclosure within the debate about two opposing models of how health is determined. Despite protestations about the need for multifactorial explanations, much social medicine work remained locked in the chains of this confrontational model. Furthermore, it was difficult then (see Rosen, 1947), and it has proved difficult since (see Stacey and Homans, 1978), to liberate social medicine from a medicine of the social; that is, to conceptualize, theorize and practise the study of the social relations of health as an activity which does not in some direct or indirect way feed off that of medicine itself. As George Rosen (1947) has argued, the lack of a theoretical base for social medicine was especially weakening. The link with the developing professionalization of social science was crucial, but sociology as distinct from social policy was in its own infancy (Halliday, 1968). One implication of this is that the history of social medicine is very largely that of social policy. This certainly makes sense from the standpoint of how Titmuss's own career subsequently developed.

In the last substantive piece he ever wrote, an account of his treatment as a cancer patient (Titmuss, 1974), Titmuss expressed the view that much of his talking and writing about social policy and social growth amounted to the observation that the most important aspects of social relations are essentially unquantifiable: they have to do with 'the texture of relationships between human beings.' This was, and is, at once the weakness and the strength of social medicine, medical sociology, and social science – all three. For the effort to translate the qualitative into the quantitative, which has dominated all sciences of the social, whether medical or not, is the basic misconception, and we are probably only now at the beginning of the path that will enable us to formulate the challenge in a different and more imaginative way (see Oakley, 1992).

Notes

1. The relevant archives include files of correspondence from 1936 to 1973, many papers and other manuscripts in draft form, 139 letters exchanged by Richard and Kathleen Titmuss during their wartime separation and 189 letters and aerographs written by Titmuss and Morris to each other while Morris was posted abroad in India. These papers are in the possession of Ann Oakley, Titmuss's daughter.

References

- Armstrong, D., *Political Anatomy of the Body* (Cambridge: Cambridge University Press, 1983).
- Bartley, M., *Authorities and Partisans: The Debate on Unemployment and Health* (Edinburgh: Edinburgh University Press, 1992).
- Caradog Jones, D., *Social Surveys* (London: Hutchinson, n.d.). Editorial, 'Social Medicine,' *British Medical Journal*, 25 July 1942, 101.
- Galton, F., *Essays in Eugenics* (London: The Eugenics Education Society, 1909).
- Grotjahn, A., *Soziale Pathologie* (3rd edition, Berlin: Springer, 1923).
- Haldane, J. B. S., *Heredity and Politics* (London: Allen and Unwin, 1938), 24–5.
- Halliday, R. J., 'The Sociological Movement, the Sociological Society and the Genesis of Academic Sociology in Britain,' *Sociological Review*, 16 (3) (1968), 377–98.
- Illsley, R., *Professional or Public Health?* (London: Nuffield Provincial Hospitals Trust, 1980).
- Jones, G., *Social Hygiene in Twentieth Century Britain* (London: Croom Helm, 1986).
- Lewis, J., *What Price Community Medicine?* (Brighton, Sussex: Wheatsheaf Books, 1986).
- Mackenzie, D., 'Eugenics in Britain,' *Social Studies of Science*, 6 (1976), 499–532.

- Morris, J. N. and Titmuss, R. M., 'Epidemiology of juvenile Rheumatism,' *Lancet,* 18 July 1942, 59–65.
- Morris, J. N. and Titmuss, R. M., 'Health and Social Change: 1.The Recent History of Rheumatic Heart Disease,' *The Medical Officer*, 26 August, 2 and 9 September (1944a).
- Morris, J. N. and Titmuss, R. M., 'Epidemiology of Peptic Ulcer: Vital Statistics,' *Lancet,* 30 December (1944b), 841–56.
- Oakley, A., 'Eugenics, Social Medicine and the Career of Richard Titmuss in Britain 1935–50,' *British Journal of Sociology*, 42 (2) (1991), 165–94.
- Oakley, A., *Social Support and Motherhood: The Natural History of a Research Project* (Oxford: Basil Blackwell, 1992).
- Oakley, A., *Man and Wife: Richard and Kay Titmuss - My Parents' Early Years* (London: Harper Collins, 1996).
- Porter, D. and Porter, R., 'What was Social Medicine? An Historiographical Essay,' *Journal of Historical Sociology*, 1 (1) (1988), 90–106.
- Problem Families Committee, *Problem Families: Six Pilot Enquiries* (London: Eugenics Society, 1948).
- Rosen, G., 'What is Social Medicine?,' *Bulletin of the History of Medicine,* 21 (1947), 674–733.
- Ryle, J. A., 'Social Medicine: its Meaning and Scope,' *British Medical Journal,* 20 November (1943).
- Searle, G. R., 'Eugenics and Politics in Britain in the 1930s,' *Annals of Science,* 35 (1979), 159–69.
- Stacey, M., *The Sociology of Health and Healing* (London: Unwin Hyman, 1988).
- Stacey, M. with Homans, H., 'The Sociology of Health and Illness: its Present State, Future Prospects and Potential for Health Research,' *Sociology*, 12 (2) (1978), 281–307.
- Teitelbaum, M. S. and Winter, J. W., *The Fear of Population Decline* (New York: Academic Press, 1985).
- Titmuss, R. M., *Poverty and Population* (London: Macmillan, 1938).
- Titmuss, R. M., *Birth, Poverty and Wealth* (London: Hamish Hamilton, 1943).
- Titmuss, R. M., *Problems of Social Policy* (London: HMSO, 1950).
- Titmuss, R. M., *Social Policy: An Introduction* (London: Allen and Unwin, 1974).
- Titmuss, R. M. and Titmuss, K., *Parents Revolt* (London: Secker and Warburg, 1942).
- Webster, C., 'Oxford and the Origins of Social Medicine,' *The Society for the Social History of Medicine Bulletin,* 38 (1986), 52– 6.

4

The Decline of Social Medicine in Britain in the 1960s

Dorothy Porter

Discipline formation has been widely studied within the history of science.[1] But little attention has so far been given to the disappearance of academic disciplines. Do disciplines die or do they simply become transformed, absorbed or transmuted? A recent example of such institutional change is the almost complete disappearance of university departments of geography in the United States.[2] Academics who have trained in geography departments do research into areas such as historical and contemporary demography and epidemiology or the spatial distribution of resources, and teach within history, sociology or other social science departments.[3] Geography divided up into so many specialisms that it eventually became absorbed into the social sciences and ceased to exist as an independent academic enterprise within what have been traditionally identified as the 'humanities' and the social sciences. A different trend is currently observable in relation to the academic study of English literature. University departments of English both in the United States and in Britain contain increasing numbers of scholars engaged in interdisciplinary studies. English, unlike geography, appears to be gradually colonizing other intellectual disciplines under a new theoretical paradigm which it vaguely refers to as 'critical theory' or 'discourse theory' grounded in a cognitive faith in 'post-modernist relativism.' Practitioners trained in and now teaching in English literature departments declare the existing disciplinary boundaries 'dead ducks' as they engage in more and more interdisciplinary research with philosophy, history and sociology.[4] The process by which academic disciplines emerge and transmute is historically complex and unique to each but commonly involves the politics of theory formation and its practical application. In this regard the institutional career of the academic discipline of social medicine offers some provocative insights. Social medicine never died, because departments continue to exist[5] and there seems to be a current trend toward creating new ones[6] in universities and medical schools both in Europe and in the United States. However, in Britain academic researchers and teachers in social medicine did lose a significant battle at the end of the 1960s which affected the discipline's influence upon future developments. At that time many departments of social medicine changed their title.[7]

I want to begin by outlining the original conceptualization of social medicine as an academic discipline in Britain and discuss the transformations it underwent during its professionalization and institutional establishment following the Second World War. I shall then examine the institutional role played by social medicine in pre- and post-graduate medical education in the period leading up to the formation of the Faculty of Community Medicine in 1972. In telling this story I hope to highlight something of the intellectual and institutional relationships between medicine and social science in Britain since the Second World War.[8]

Political Positivism

At a conference held on 2 April 1965 by the Society for Social Medicine, Thomas McKeown,[9] Professor of Social Medicine at Birmingham University since 1945, emphasized the separate identity of social medicine as an academic discipline from its association with the humanitarian tradition in medicine.[10]

> Since it came into general use in Britain some twenty-five years ago the term social medicine has been used in two very different ways: as an expression of the humanitarian tradition in medicine; and as a name for an academic discipline. The first usage is general and imprecise, and our concern here will be with the second.

But initially the conceptualization of social medicine as an academic discipline was vigorously linked to humanitarian politics.[11]

Just after the first British Professor of Social Medicine, John Ryle, retired in 1949, McKeown wrote to him expressing deep regret at this loss to the profession. McKeown acknowledged Ryle as the founder of the discipline and the pioneer of its institutional establishment.[12] Their perceptions of social medicine and its function differed in an important way. For Ryle social medicine was an ideological mission with a political purpose and a social responsibility.[13] It was also the heir-apparent to clinical medicine and would change the role of medicine in society by deconstructing medicine at the bedside. Social physicians would practise whole-person medicine in place of technologically determined specialists steeped in the epistemological orthodoxies of experimental science. Doctors trained in social medicine would fulfil their true Hippocratic destiny by becoming naturalist interpreters of health and disease and teachers of a new creed to society. That creed was what Ryle's contemporary Julian Huxley had identified as 'scientific humanism.'[14] For Ryle the 'social conscience and scientific intent' of social medicine would help to establish scientific humanism as a new secular ethic governing social, economic and political behaviour, and he stressed that 'the ideas and tasks of social medicine may be justly regarded as essential contributions (perhaps the most essential and practical of any at present within our range) to the developing philosophy of scientific humanism.'[15] This function, Ryle insisted, did not constitute a form of party politics. It was, instead, the foundation upon which political decision-making could be based. For Ryle scientific humanism went beyond party politics because its aim was the corporate management of human welfare. Designing an 'equality of opportunity for health' was one of its tasks. Assisting the establishment of a religion of rationalism in a new social order was another.[16]

Social medicine in Britain in the 1940s aimed to become a medicine of society for society. Emerging from the politics of science and ethics, its mission was to facilitate progressive human social and biological evolution. As an expression of scientific humanism social medicine was to be part of the rising tide of corporate welfarism. John Ryle believed that this could be achieved by changing clinical medicine into a new discipline of holistic socio-biology of health and disease. The new discipline was grounded in holistic epistemology and a deeply confirmed rejection of mechanistic positivism. Before Ryle died, however, positivism in the form of highly quantitative research into population health already began to dominate the discipline. *The British Journal of Social Medicine* was founded and edited by Francis Crew and Lancelot Hogben in 1947 and was dedicated to analysing the 'numerical, structural and functional changes of human populations in their biological and medical aspects.'[17] The editors suggested that the methods of social medicine 'must necessarily be statistical, involving the use of numerical data obtained either from official sources or from special field investigations, and interpreted in the light of established findings of the laboratory and of the clinic.'[18]

The positivist orientation of the new journal was not surprising given its editorship. Hogben was an avowed opponent of 'holism' which he viewed as self-indulgent mysticism by privileged intellectuals who did not have to think about the practical ways in which science could engender social change.[19] Hogben believed that mechanistic, positivist science was emancipatory. He linked his epistemology of science to his political philosophy of socialism. Facts, proofs, knowledge could promote social change. Science could build a new society because it offered objective truth. He opposed the 'holistic' Marxism of some of his socialist-scientific associates in the 1930s, such as J. B. S. Haldane. Occasionally this difference of opinion blew up into a full-scale scholarly row, as it had done with his friend, the biologist Joseph Needam.[20]

Hogben and Crew had long been associated in research into animal genetics, comparative physiology, and human ecology and population genetics. They shared a positivist philosophy of science and a cognitive enthusiasm for the power of statistical methods and explanations. Their association had begun when Crew appointed Hogben Deputy Director of his Animal Breeding Research Department at Edinburgh University in 1921. Hogben characterized the Department as keeping alive the British interest in chromosome research after the First World War. Consequently it attracted those few British biologists interested in genetics and experimentalism. After a summer-long visit to the Department by J. B. S. Haldane and Julian Huxley, they and Crew and Hogben founded the *British Journal of Experimental Biology* and the Society of Experimental Biology in 1924.[21] Given Crew's pioneering role in the support of genetic science in Britain, Hogben suggested that the only reason he decided to leave it and enter into the new discipline of social medicine following the Second World War was that the term 'social medicine' implied 'human ecology.' Hogben describes Crew's decision to leave genetic research as 'fateful' coming after a 'period of deep mental anguish.'[22]

> When he undertook onerous responsibilities in connection with the official history of army medicine during World War II, Crew, like most of us, lived from day to day in a miasma of uncertainty about what the future held. When Sidney Smith offered him in 1944 the Edinburgh Chair of Public Health and Social Medicine, he must have realised how Herculean was the task to which he had committed himself as part editor, part author of the official history. Had he decided to return to his first love, he would have had to

> abandon a pedestrian undertaking from which what many of his admirers might well regard as a misguided sense of loyalty prevented his escape.

Such a loss to genetic science could only be justified, Hogben suggested, by the inclusion of human ecology into the old academic discipline of public health. 'In the view of those who promoted the change from "Public Health", hitherto conceived primarily in terms of epidemiology, to "Public Health and Social Medicine", human ecology was what the addition of the last two words implied. At least, one charitably may believe this to be so.'[23] Indeed, Crew did perceive the hereditary basis to population health as crucial. He identified the true father of the modern academic study of social medicine as Alfred Grotjahn who founded his theory of social hygiene on the eugenic concept of social pathology.[24] But Crew believed that both heredity and environment equally determined health and was emphatic that the new discipline must be based upon a marriage between the social and biological sciences, both of which were dependent upon quantitative analysis. But this would change the social role of medicine. Traditionally,[25]

> the shape of medicine has in the past ever been a reflection of the shape of the society of which it was a part. It is now being given the opportunity of playing a notable role in changing the shape of that society, of initiating a change and not merely reflecting it.

Medicine could realize this new role by embracing the social sciences because Crew believed that their function was to bring about social change and promote social amelioration.[26]

> Medicine is not as yet sufficiently prepared to play its full part in ... social amelioration and human betterment. Its development as a social science is not yet sufficiently advanced. The rate of this development must be accelerated.

Social medicine must bring about the evolution of medicine as a science of social amelioration through an integrated intellectual programme examining all aspects of 'human and social biology and human ecology.'[27] In this way medicine could realize its contribution towards social reform providing 'information of a scientific kind which can form the basis of action relating to social amelioration.'[28] But for Crew the methodological base or the 'investigational instruments of social medicine' were 'biostatistics and field investigational teams. By means of these, records are collected and the knowledge contained within them is distilled.' Social medicine was forced to rely on such analytical tools because 'the human animal cannot be used deliberately as experimental material in a controlled environment' but instead 'he is unique in that records of his behaviour can be and are maintained.' Statistical analysis could substitute for experimental logic as the scientific basis of 'the therapy of social medicine' which was not medical but 'social and political action based upon medical recommendation.'[29]

In the *British Journal of Preventive and Social Medicine* Crew and Hogben separated politically orientated research from the politics of medical organization as a whole: 'This Journal is not meant to provide a platform for those who wish to present their views concerning the place of social medicine in the organisational set-up of medicine as a whole.'[30] Social medicine may have been conceived of as a transforming influence by its founders such as Ryle and Crew but not within the conventional context of medical administration and organization. The idea that the politics of social reform could be best served through the pursuit of ground-breaking research within the context of academic science was to continue to guide the institutional development of the discipline in the following decade.

This was central to the agenda set for the institutionalization of social medicine by Thomas McKeown. McKeown succeeded Crew and Hogben as editor of the *British Journal of Social Medicine*. After the death of Ryle and the retirement of Crew and William Hobson at Sheffield, he also became the longest-standing professor of social medicine in Britain and a dominating figure within the discipline. McKeown shared, with Crew and Hogben, a belief in the emancipatory power of positivist science and socialist politics. Hogben, who spent some of the latter years of his career at Birmingham, had a direct influence upon him. Like Crew and Hogben he remained wedded to a faith in the force of quantitative explanations.

McKeown's mission for social medicine included discrediting the triumphalist myths of clinical medicine. He used an historical-quantitative analysis to argue that improvements in health and 'the modern rise of population' resulted from increased nutrition, higher standards of living and public health measures. Advances in clinical medicine and therapeutic methods had come too late and affected too small a proportion of the population to have played a role in the extension of average length of life and mortality decline amongst twentieth-century affluent societies. His destruction of some of the pretensions of technologically advanced medicine aimed to justify the primacy of the role of social medicine in providing society with what Crew had described as 'political therapies' for population health. McKeown shared a common vision with Crew and Hogben of the relationship between science and socialism, but the environment in which he pursued it changed after the war when professional and academic politics became crucial.

Counting on Health and the Creation of the Community Physician: Academic Research and the Practice of Service Provision

In 1942 the Royal College of Physicians set up a committee to investigate the role that 'Social and Preventive Medicine' should play in medical education. The Committee clearly distinguished social from preventive medicine.[31]

> Social Medicine is concerned with the social environment and with heredity in so far as these affect health and well being. Preventive Medicine is more executive in outlook and comprises the design and direction of measures for the preservation of health and the prevention of disease.

Crew commented in 1949 that the conception of social medicine represented in the Reports of both this and the Interdepartmental Committee on Medical Education (the *Goodenough Report*, 1944) was pretty narrow and inadequate. Nevertheless the identity of social medicine as an academic discipline of pure research, as a separate intellectual enterprise from training in the practical art of service administration and management, structured its subsequent institutionalization and professionalization.

The hopes for rapid academic institutionalization of social medicine articulated in the 1940s were not met following the war. After Ryle died in 1950, for example, his chair at the Institute of Social Medicine, Oxford was not renewed and his successor as director, Alice Stewart, remained a university Reader. The institutionalization of the discipline did expand until in 1956 there was a sufficient number of researchers and university teachers in the field in Britain to form a learned society, the Society for Social Medicine. Earlier that year the Society of Medical Officers of Health had decided to set up a new division for academic teachers of preventive medicine but membership would be restricted to those who were medically qualified. When the president of the SMOH, Sir Selwyn Selwyn-Clarke, wrote[32] about these proposals to Thomas McKeown, he responded by suggesting that an independent society was needed which allowed medical and non-medical academics to focus on research in social medicine.[33]

> I think there is no doubt that the objects of this body will differ substantially from those of the group which the Executive Committee of the SMOH is contemplating. To mention two points of difference, the society will be concerned mainly with research, and original papers will occupy most of the time at its meetings, and membership will not be restricted to those with medical or dental qualifications.

McKeown was clearly doubtful about the plans of the SMOH:[34]

> Whether a group of teachers associated with the SMOH would also serve a useful purpose I feel less qualified to judge .... However, I would have thought that the objects of the group should be considered carefully in the light of the creation of the new society.

The Society was subsequently set up on a basis of restricted and invitation-only membership in order to maintain its academic character.[35]

The need to separate the research-based academic discipline from the practical concerns of service provision continued to be a common goal amongst the Society's membership. A decade after its foundation the membership was still only 150 but all were engaged in either full-time research or teaching social medicine. As the Society's secretary informed M. R. Draper, the Deputy Registrar of the GMC, in 1964, 'Consequently, most of us are either members of university departments of social medicine, public health, epidemiology and medical statistics or of establishments engaged in epidemiological or medical care research.'[36]

Nevertheless the intellectual scope and institutional role of the discipline remained indeterminate. This was highlighted when the Society came to give evidence firstly to the GMC's Committee on Medical Education set up in 1964 and then to the Royal Commission on Medical Education set up under the chairmanship of Lord Todd in 1966. As mentioned above, the Society held a conference in April 1965 to plan its submission. Thomas McKeown gave a talk which attempted to define the parameters and role of the discipline.[37]

> It is now approximately 22 or 23 years since Professor Ryle went to Oxford and it may seem surprising that it is still necessary to discuss at some length what is meant by social medicine, not only in respect of the medical public at large, but even among teachers themselves.

But even confining definitions to what was taught as social medicine was insufficient because 'At the present time it is particularly important to consider more than just the question of what the departments teach.'[38] He was sure, however, that two traditional features endured, 'the approach to medical problems by population methods and the interest in the medical needs of society.'[39] So for McKeown the mission to address the social relations of health was linked to the quantitative analysis of them. This was the important legacy which social medicine inherited from public health. Up to the mid-nineteenth century public health had approached what was insoluble on an individual basis by analysing the 'population point of view.'[40] This directed medicine towards its social responsibilities.[41]

> I am not suggesting that this was because the people who started all of this were very wise and had seen ahead as to what would be likely to be required in future. I think these were inescapable features of the early movement which was inevitably focused on the infectious diseases. There wasn't any approach which wasn't population based and there had to be public developments to deal with the threat of infectious diseases.

McKeown argued that despite the epidemiological transition from predominantly infectious to chronic disease in 'developed countries'[42] the 'population approach' remained linked, indeed, inevitably led medicine to engage with its essential social function, the organization of society's needs regarding the promotion of health and the reduction of sickness. Quantitative socio-medical analysis was thus an inherently political activity. In this sense McKeown reflected the earlier 'political' positivism of Lancelot Hogben whom he greatly admired.[43]

McKeown insisted that the social function of social medicine was bound to the prosecution of research. Teaching was a secondary concern. The research produced by the discipline would be the persuasive factor not only for establishing intellectual credibility and political force but also for acquiring institutional security.[44]

> For a medical school which hasn't yet got a department the thing doesn't present in the form of whether to teach such and such. It presents in the form of do we have reason to introduce a full-time department, and the reasons for doing that are very largely to do with research as well as teaching.

McKeown believed that a full-time department of social medicine should occupy the same relation to the medical school as a university department of physiology. Knowledge and methods of the subject would be taught to medical students based on the innovative research which defined the discipline. And the correct description of social medical research was the application of 'population methods' – by which he meant medical, epidemiological and demographic statistics – to three broad fields, human biology, human disease, and medicine in society. He stressed that this definition did not conflate the meaning of social medicine with epidemiology.[45]

> Some people identify academic social medicine with epidemiology, which they conceive to be concerned only with the study of disease. If this restriction is accepted for epidemiology – and we hope it will not be – there are reasons for not accepting it for social medicine.

McKeown echoed Ryle's concerns with the study of the 'normal' by insisting that 'Except sometimes in the field of infectious disease, investigation of the "abnormal" requires the support of observations on the "normal".'[46] Social medicine in this sense was still a Rylean 'hygiology' or science of health.

While all of these areas, human biology, human disease and medicine in society, were legitimate subjects for research through population analysis, a social medicine department should largely focus on researching and teaching the latter. Social medicine should contribute to both the pre-clinical and clinical teaching of the two former subjects – possibly through joint classes – and the analysis of medicine in society should be the sole responsibility of social medicine at either a pre- or post-graduate level.[47] McKeown wanted to differentiate social medicine as much as possible from the clinical agenda. The task of social medicine research and teaching must be to insure that 'in future doctors are better acquainted with the nature of the medical task, and understand the complexity of the setting in which it must be tackled.'[48] This did not, however, require the methods of medical sociology as far as McKeown was concerned who thought that, while there might be room for it in the realm of research, it had no place in the medical curriculum.[49]

At the conference itself McKeown's paper stimulated considerable debate. Some of his colleagues in the Society believed that social medicine should be restricted to epidemiology alone and agreed that medical sociology should be limited to a pre-medical subject.[50] Others such as Alwyn Smith, Margot Jefferys and Marvin Susser believed that the sociology of institutions and the social determinants of illness behaviour, recovery and aetiology should be essential components of medical education.[51] Others were anxious that social medicine should not isolate itself from clinical medicine but should overcome divisions and intellectual prejudices between medical disciplines.[52]

Despite these disputes and after extensive effort by the Society to explore all avenues, the final submission of evidence to the Royal Commission bore remarkable resemblance to McKeown's original rough-drafted conference paper. Some significant changes were made, however. In the submission the scope of social medicine was now defined by the Society as consisting of '(a) epidemiology and (b) the study of the medical needs of society.'[53] Epidemiology was considered 'in our interpretation' to mean 'the application of population methods to problems of human biology as well as of human disease.'[54] Also the Society now suggested that the investigation of disease determinants required observation of 'anatomical, physiological and sociological variables.' The Society collectively stated that[55]

> It follows that research in social medicine is concerned with the application of statistical and sociological methods to the study of human biology and human disease and of medical and related services.

The Society also believed that academic departments of social medicine should have research and teaching responsibilities for a number of related subjects such as medical statistics, human genetics – at least population rather than molecular-biological genetics – and various branches of the behavioural sciences such as the social psychology of health and illness and the evaluation of services.[56]

Like McKeown's original paper the Society's submission emphasized that the only undergraduate teaching which a department should be solely responsible for was the analysis of medicine in society, which consisted of a few basic themes: the current state of community health and its determinants; the effects upon the community of changes in size, age structure and genetic constitution of the population; epidemiology of major diseases; the evolution of medical services, their current organization, and possibilities for improvement.[57]

With regard to postgraduate education the Society expressed dissatisfaction with the inadequacies of the Diploma in Public Health as a qualification for various branches of medical administration beyond the appointment of a medical officer of health.[58] The GMC then asked the Society to submit further evidence to their special committee set up later in 1966 on post-graduate education in public health.[59] The numbers registering for the DPH had fallen dramatically. Various medical administrators, such as hospital SMAOs, had expressed exasperation with the current system of qualification. This time the Society used the opportunity to suggest that the DPH had become redundant, orientated as it was to an administrative post which had more relevance to nineteenth- rather than twentieth-century British society. They suggested that it be replaced by a broader-based course which would serve the purposes of postgraduate students pursuing numerous different career paths in medical and health service administration.[60] From the submissions of the Society to both the GMC and the Todd commission it is clear that academic departments in social medicine aspired to be university research faculties with special responsibilities for undergraduate medical education and a monopoly on postgraduate education for service workers.[61]

The report of the Royal Commission – the *Todd Report*[62] – was published the following year. One of the most significant of its recommendations was that a new professional body should be created which would draw together the wide variety of professionals who worked in preventive medicine or the administration of medical services. The new professional organization would also be responsible for regulating a new specialist qualification in what the Report identified as 'community medicine.'[63]

> In Community Medicine there is a great need for a professional body which can bring together all the interests, academic and service, and which has the support and strength to undertake the assessment needed during and at the end of general professional training.

The term 'community medicine' described an intellectual union between academic social medicine and practical service provision and it became increasingly popular. In 1969 the Royal Institute of Public Health and Hygiene renamed its journal *Community Health* in order to address 'What is Public Health and Hygiene in the Seventies?'[64] By 1970 a Government Green Paper[65] which explored the future reorganization of the National Health Service began using the term 'community physician' to replace the medical officer of health. John Pemberton, Professor of Social and Preventive Medicine at Queen's Belfast, wrote to Molly Newhouse, the Honorary Secretary of the Society in April 1969,[66] that in the light of the *Todd Report* the GMC was going to set up a speciality board in 'public health, social medicine, community medicine or whatever it is going to be called.' The important thing as far as the Society members were concerned was that 'the academic side of our subject ... should be well represented in the preliminary discussions.' Pemberton envisaged a sort of college of community medicine being created but the problem would be how to integrate the academic –

consisting of university departments of social medicine – and applied branches – i.e. public health medical officers, hospital medical administrators, etc.– of the profession into one faculty. Pemberton thought that the idea which had been floated of creating a new faculty within the Royal College of Physicians might be one solution but only if it did not disbar those without sufficient qualifications to enter the College itself. He wondered if some MOHs would be eligible for membership. Nevertheless he felt these new developments should become a priority concern of the Society, which must find a means to 'bring the academic and applied sides together and to try and create a coherent speciality for the future.'[67]

Informal discussions between various groups had begun in 1968 concerning the possibility of setting up a new faculty. The group included representatives from the Royal Colleges, the School itself, the Society for Social Medicine, the Society of Medical Officers of Health and representatives from various medical and health administrators' associations who eventually formed a formal working party in the autumn of 1969. The group had already outlined a number of basic principles, however, at a meeting at the London School of Hygiene and Tropical Medicine in May 1969.[68] They agreed that a new Faculty of Community Medicine be set up under the auspices of the Royal Colleges of Physicians which would embrace 'those engaged in Community Medicine and Epidemiology.'[69] The group, at this stage, suggested that membership would include 'both those qualified in medicine and also non-medical experts who play an increasingly important part in medicine.'[70] Furthermore, examination would not be the only means of entry to the Faculty but it would 'be responsible for setting its own standards, and organising its own examinations and training programmes.'[71]

The Society elected two representatives, Richard Doll and Jerry Morris, to serve on the Working Party. But from the outset some Society members were sceptical about the value of a new Faculty for academics rather than practitioners of community medicine. McKeown wrote to Richard Doll in April 1969 expressing the doubts of members of his own department at Birmingham:[72]

> There would be considerable resentment of a professional organisation for social medicine which excluded non-medical statisticians, epidemiologists etc. My colleagues would therefore favour either of two approaches: (a) a professional organisation of medical administrators which might include a few academics who had trained as administrators, but would exclude the Dolls, Casses

and McKeowns as well as the Headys and Waterhouses; or (b) a professional organisation concerned with social medicine which would include both medical and non-medical people with varied backgrounds. The second possibility is unlikely to be feasible under the RCP.

As negotiations about the proposed Faculty continued, further dissent appeared amongst the membership of the Society for Social Medicine. Some members believed that the title of any new organization should continue to be Social Medicine and that the term Community Medicine would give priority to service training and under-represent academic research in the subject. Alwyn Smith, by this time Professor of Preventive and Social Medicine at Manchester, wrote directly to the Registrar of the Royal College of Physicians in May 1970.[73] An informal group of 'Heads of Departments of Social Medicine in the Midlands' circulated a letter to other departmental heads throughout Britain and Ireland to gather opinion from which 'a clear-cut consensus' emerged.[74] Smith identified two major objections which all but John Pemberton agreed with. Firstly,[75]

> The title 'Community Medicine' is misleading. The word 'community' frequently has a connotation which excludes hospitals and the expression Community Medicine, in other parts of the English speaking world, is often synonymous with General Practice. We believe that 'Social Medicine' would be the best for a Faculty but there would be some support for the alternatives of 'Social and Preventive Medicine,' or 'Social Medicine and Public Health' .

Smith emphasized the strong concern of his colleagues that their opinion should carry significant weight in terms of the negotiations surrounding the Faculty.[76]

> The full-time academic Departments of Social Medicine have a special concern in relation to the formation of any such Faculty since they are concerned with the training of recruits to all branches of its discipline as well as for the recruitment and training of both medical and non-medical academic staff. We therefore feel strongly that the Heads of full-time Departments of Social Medicine should have their views strongly directed to the Colleges of Physicians.

The Society's representatives on the Working Party were disturbed by this intervention but continued to participate in negotiations.[77] As these continued, however, the original principles of non-medical eligibility and qualification for Faculty membership were lost. The Society members saw less and less advantage for them in the creation of the new Faculty under the terms now proposed.[78]

At an Extraordinary General Meeting of the Society in January 1971 members began to question the benefit of the whole enterprise.[79] Many of the Society's members would be excluded from the Faculty under the new terms of entry and thus academic social medicine would be vastly under-represented. Furthermore, if the Faculty set up its own specialist registration the academic departments would be significantly controlled by its actions without being able to influence its decision-making. Archie Cochrane expressed the sense of the meeting when he 'queried what the Royal Colleges were actually offering.'[80] A discussion ensued which concluded that 'apart from some contact between different branches of medicine, there was little self-evident benefit.'[81] The Society then voted on whether to continue to participate in the process of setting up a new Faculty or whether to withdraw altogether. On balance the meeting was persuaded by Richard Doll's point that to exempt themselves from the negotiation process would leave the Society powerless to influence events.[82]

In the autumn of 1971, however, the AGM of the Society directed its chairman, George Knox, to write directly to Lord Cohen, the president of the GMC, expressing their reservations about the direction of events. The central issue was that[83]

> The Society was concerned that the Colleges might apply for an effective monopoly of conditions necessary for specialist registration.

The DPH had traditionally been under the control of university departments, within the context of the regulations set down by the GMC. But[84]

> Faculty proposals which pre-empted the design of courses and training schemes through a unilateral declaration of training or examination requirements would be unacceptable to the University departments.

Furthermore the Society would not accept any new specialist registration procedure which required the payment of annual fees to the Royal Colleges. But more than anything else the Society was concerned that a Faculty-controlled qualification would result in imposing an 'educational stereotype.'[85] Knox pointed out to Cohen that 'Social Medicine, or Community Medicine as it is called in the

Todd Report' was a broad and diverse field with many subspecialities.[86] The Todd Commission believed that these diverse groups should be brought together but nevertheless any successful attempt must 'recognise this diversity in designing training schemes and career pathways. A single educational pathway would be a danger which, if carried beyond the preliminary stages, could not reach the high standards needed in every part of the field.'[87]

But the concerns of academics in social medicine were overshadowed by the joint goals of the Royal Colleges and the physicians who worked in the public health service. Both wanted to offer the opportunity for consultant status in preventive medicine, which became the prime objective of the terms under which the new Faculty was eventually established. The new Faculty was dominated therefore by what Pemberton had called the 'applied side' of the discipline, i.e. community physicians involved in service provision. As a result the creation of the new Faculty and later a new office of Community Physician to replace the old MOH legitimated the rise of a new discipline, community medicine, with its focus on the practical concerns of service planning and management.[88] Academic departments of social medicine ultimately had to adapt to the new world of community medicine, even, in some cases, changing their name – as did the first Institute of Social Medicine at Oxford which was transformed into a Department of Social and Community Medicine. The disarray in community medicine itself by the end of the 1980s stimulated yet further debate. Ironically the Acheson report of 1988 highlighted the need to bring back public health into the concept of prevention.[89]

Conclusion

Social medicine did not die as an academic discipline but its intellectual parameters and institutional scope dramatically changed during its academic professionalization and eventually it was overtaken by events in the late 1960s. The allegiance of the discipline to a model of pure research eventually left it ill-equipped to cope with the politics of service provision which it exempted itself from as it became institutionalized within a university setting.

John Ryle, Francis Crew and Thomas McKeown had all conceived of the marriage of medicine and the social sciences as a political mission dedicated to the improvement of society through direct influence on policy-making and execution. But unlike Ryle, Crew and McKeown believed that the political mission of social medicine was bound to a positivistic model of knowledge.

Quantitative social scientific research would determine its political role, providing the basis for its reform mission. McKeown believed that research could only be supported through institutional establishment and this became a dominant concern during the period of professionalization in the 1950s and 1960s. Concern to enhance intellectual rigour by separating research and teaching from the practical concerns of service provision, however, led to increasing isolation of academic departments of social medicine from the policy-making process. The price to pay for this division was a failure to negotiate the health service reorganization of the late 1960s and early 1970s which bought off the now-redundant service providers with spurious academic status and honours. Community medicine gave former Medical Officers of Health a new intellectual and practical identity in health service management and allowed the 1974 reorganization to go ahead without the potential obstacle of their opposition.

The isolation of social medicine was enhanced by the fact that its epistemological agenda narrowed. The study of 'population health and disease' was vastly reduced in scope from the holistic union of theory and practice in the establishment of scientific humanism as a new social ethic. As social medicine developed in Britain after the Second World War the influence of social science became limited to the empirical methods of quantitative social research. The theoretical explosion of the post-war social sciences barely influenced the quantitative model of social-medical analysis. Nevertheless the growth of the discipline kept the opportunity for interaction between medicine and social science open, but yet another new discipline began to enter this field. That was, of course, the social scientific sub-speciality, medical sociology. The relationship of social medicine to medical sociology, however, is another story which is pursued in further detail throughout this volume.

Notes

1. See for example the history of molecular biology presented in Robert C. Olby, *The Path to the Double Helix* (London: Macmillan, 1974).
2. See *The World of Learning* (London: Europa, 1995).
3. See for example the contributions on historical demography by geographers to *The Journal of Interdisciplinary History* and *Social History of Medicine* over the last ten years.
4. See for example *Speculum, Representations* and *Paragraph: The Journal of the Modern Critical Theory Group.*
5. For example, the Department of Social Medicine at Birmingham.
6. For example, the Department of Epidemiology at Bristol University changed its name to the Department of Social Medicine in 1995.
7. For example, the Department of Social Medicine at Oxford became the Department of Social and Community Medicine in the 1970s.
8. See also Margot Jefferys, 'The Transition from Public Health to Community Medicine: The Evolution and Execution of a Policy for Occupational Transformation,' *Bulletin of the Society for the Social History of Medicine*, 39 (1986), 47–63; *idem*, 'Social Science Teaching in Medical Education: An Overview of the Situation in Great Britain,' in Magdalen Sokolowska *et al.* (eds), *Health, Medicine, Society* (Boston: D. Reidel, 1973); *idem*, 'Serendipity: An Autobiographical Account of the Career of a Medical Sociologist in Britain,' in R. H. Elling and M. Sokolowska (eds), *Medical Sociologists at Work* (New Brunswick, N.J.: Transactions Press, 1978), 135–61; *idem*, 'Does Medicine Need Sociology?,' in D. Tuckett and J. M. Kaufert (eds), *Basic Readings in Medical Sociology* (London: Tavistock Publications 1978); *idem*, 'Social Science and Medical Education in Britain: A Sociological Analysis of their Relationship,' *International Journal of Health Services*, 4 (1974), 549–63; Leo William Simmons, *Social Science in Medicine* (New York: Russell Sage Foundation, 1954); Margaret Reid, 'The Development of Medical Sociology in Britain' (Discussion Papers in Social Research, University of Glasgow, 1975–6).
9. Thomas McKeown, *Lancet*, ii (1988), 58; *British Medical Journal*, 297 (1988), 129.

10. Thomas McKeown, 'Social Medicine as an Academic Discipline,' first draft paper for the Society for the Social History of Medicine. Special one-day conference on 'Social Medicine in the Medical Curriculum' [held at LSHTM, 2 April 1965], private collection of papers, from now on referred to as McKeown, 'First Draft.' The records of the conference itself with the papers and discussions of the speakers: T. McKeown, J. N. Morris, E. M. Backett, C. R. Lowe, J. Knowelden, are in the *Archives of the Society for Social Medicine* held at the *Contemporary Medical Archives Centre*, Wellcome Institute for the History of Medicine [from now referred to as *SA/SSM*], *SA/SSM, A, 19.*
11. *Ibid.*
12. McKeown to Ryle, 1 February 1950. [J.A. Ryle, *Private Papers.* Held by his son, Anthony Ryle.]
13. Dorothy Porter, 'John Ryle: Doctor of Revolution?,' in Dorothy Porter and Roy Porter (eds), *Doctors, Politics and Society: Historical Essays* (Amsterdam: Rodopi, 1993), 229–47.
14. Dorothy Porter, 'Social Medicine and the New Society: Medicine and Scientific Humanism in mid-Twentieth Century Britain,' *Journal of Historical Sociology*, 9 (1996), 168–87.
15. John A. Ryle, 'Social Medicine: Its Meaning and Its Scope,' *British Medical Journal*, ii (1943), 633–6, 636.
16. John Ryle, *Fears May Be Liars* (London: Allen and Unwin, 1941).
17. 'Notice to Contributors,' *The British Journal of Social and Preventive Medicine*, 1 (1) (January, 1947), edited by F. A. E. Crew and Lancelot Hogben.
18. *Ibid.*
19. Gary Werskey, *The Visible College* (London: Allen Lane, 1978).
20. *Ibid.*
21. See Pnina Abir-Am, 'The Biotheoretical Gathering, Transdisciplinary Authority and the Incipient Legitimation of Molecular Biology in the 1930s: New Perspective on the Historical Sociology of Science,' *History of Science*, 25 (1987), 1–70.
22. Lancelot Hogben, 'Francis Albert Eley Crew, 1886–1973,' *Biographical Memoirs of the Fellows of the Royal Society*, 20 (1974), 135–53, 144.
23. *Ibid.*, 144.

24. Paul Weindling, *Health, Race and German Politics Between National Unification and Nazism 1870–1945* (Cambridge: Cambridge University Press, 1989); F. A. E. Crew, 'Social Medicine as an Academic Discipline,' in Arthur Massey, *Modern Trends in Public Health* (London: Butterworth, 1949), 62–5.
25. *Ibid.*, Crew, 47.
26. *Ibid.*, 77.
27. *Ibid.*, 78.
28. *Ibid.*
29. *Ibid.*, 77.
30. *Ibid.*
31. Quoted by Crew, *ibid.*, 69.
32. Sir Selwyn-Clarke to Thomas McKeown, 30 September 1956, *SA/SSM, A1.*
33. Thomas McKeown to Sir Selwyn-Clarke, 1 October 1956, *SA/SSM, A1.*
34. *Ibid.*
35. See 'Draft Proposal for Setting Up a Society,' following a conference organized by the British members of the International Corresponding Club (Preventive and Social Medicine) held at the CIBA Foundation 30 June –1 July 1956. *SA/SSM, A1;* see also 'J. M. Mackintosh to John Pemberton [Professor of Social Medicine at Queen's University, Belfast]. 4th July 1956.
    Dear Pemberton.
    Here is a draft informal note of the decision of the Committee on Saturday afternoon.
    "It was agreed in principle that a British Society of Preventive and Social Medicine should be formed with the following essential features: it should be a wholly independent society; its main object should be the advancement of academic social medicine, primarily in the research field; that the Society should normally hold its meetings at the various academic and research institutes with which its members are professionally associated. The place of meeting should be selected for its scientific interest rather than for accessibility. The Society should approach the governing body of the Journal of Social and Preventive Medicine with a view to forming a close association. The membership of the Society should be limited by certain criteria which will be gradually established as it develops. In the initial stages however membership would be offered to

all who hold academic and research positions in this field." *SA/SSM, A1.*

36. Margot Jefferys to M. R. Draper, Deputy Registrar, GMC, 23 December 1964, *SA/SSM, C2.*
37. Thomas McKeown, 'Social Medicine as an Academic Discipline,' final draft of conference paper given on 2 April 1964 for the Society of Social Medicine. *SA/SSM, A19*, 1, from now on referred to as McKeown, 'Final Draft.'
38. *Ibid.*, 2.
39. McKeown, 'First Draft,' *op.cit.* (ref. 10).
40. McKeown, 'Final Draft,' *op.cit.* (ref. 37), 3.
41. *Ibid.*
42. McKeown, 'First Draft,' *op.cit.* (ref. 10), 1.
43. McKeown to Jessop, 1 October 1956:
    'I think it is of special importance not to leave out senior people who, although not actually in the subject, are closely concerned with it, and whose opinions we should certainly hear. I am thinking of people like Bradford Hill, Lancelot Hogben and Aubrey Lewis.
    Yours sincerely, McKeown.' *SA/SSM, A1.*
44. *Ibid.*
45. McKeown, 'First Draft,' *op.cit.* (ref. 10), 2.
46. *Ibid.*
47. *Ibid.*, 3–4.
48. *Ibid.*, 5.
49. 'Conference Report,' *SA/SSM, A19*, 2.
50. *Ibid.*, 5. E.g. Macdonald, Reid, Acheson.
51. *Ibid.*
52. *Ibid.*, 6. E.g. Acheson, Case, Reid, Jessop.
53. Society for Social Medicine, 'Evidence to be Submitted to the Royal Commission on Medical Education,' Final Draft, unpublished manuscript, *SA/SSM, C4*, 1.
54. *Ibid.*
55. *Ibid.*, 2.
56. *Ibid.*, 7–12.
57. *Ibid.*, 4–5.
58. *Ibid.*, 5.
59. M. R. Draper to Secretary of the Society for Social Medicine, 1 April 1966, *SA/SSM, C3.*
60. Society for Social Medicine, 'Evidence to the General Medical Council's Special Committee on Public Health, 24th October, 1966,' *Private Collection of Papers*; see also 'Evidence to be

Submitted to Commission on Medical Education,' Final Draft, *op.cit.* (ref. 53), 5–6.

61. See also the Society's drafts and final submission of 'Evidence Submitted to the Working Party on Medical Administrators,' set up by Sir George E. Godber, Chief Medical Officer of the Department of Health and Social Security, in 1972. 'Draft,' *SA/SSM, C5*; published as Society for Social Medicine, 'Evidence Submitted to the Working Party on Medical Administrators,' *British Journal of Preventive and Social Medicine*, 26 (1972), 62–6. See also M. R. Alderson (Honorary Secretary, Society for Social Medicine) to Sir George E. Godber, 31 July 1972, *SA/SSM, C5.*
62. Great Britain, House of Commons, *Royal Commission on Medical Education, 1965–68. Report of the Chairman A.R. Todd* (London: HMSO, 1969), Cmnd 3569.
63. *Ibid.*, para. 138.
64. 'Editorial,' *Community Health*, 1 (6) (1969–70), 295–7.
65. *Ibid.*
66. John Pemberton to Molly Newhouse, 19 April 1969, *Private Collection of Papers.*
67. *Ibid.*
68. 'Summary of a Discussion Held to Consider the Setting up of a Faculty of Community Medicine on 1st May 1969 at 2.00p.m.,' *SA/SSM, C4.*
69. *Ibid.*, 2.
70. *Ibid.*
71. *Ibid.*
72. McKeown to Richard Doll, 16 April 1969, *SA/SSM, C14.*
73. Alwyn Smith to 'The Registrar' at the Royal College of Physicians, 6 May 1970, *Private Collection of Papers.*
74. *Ibid.*
75. *Ibid.*
76. *Ibid.*
77. See Molly Newhouse to Hubert Cambell, 21 May 1970, *SA/SSM, C14.*
78. See 'Minutes Extraordinary General Meeting of the Society for Social Medicine held at the Royal Society of Medicine, 1 Wimpole Street on 4th June, 1970,' *Private Collection of Papers.*
79. 'Minutes of the Extraordinary General Meeting of the Society for Social Medicine held at the London School of Hygiene on Saturday, 30th January, 1971 at 2.30pm,' *Private Collection of Papers.*

80. *Ibid.*, 2.
81. *Ibid.*
82. *Ibid.*, 2–3.
83. E. G. Knox to Lord Cohen, 'Copy of Letter Sent to President of the General Medical Council Following the Annual General Meeting, 1971,' *Private Collection of Papers*, 1.
84. *Ibid.*, 2.
85. *Ibid.*
86. *Ibid.*
87. *Ibid.*
88. See Jane Lewis, *What Price Community Medicine? The Philosophy, Practice and Politics of Public Health Since 1919* (Brighton: Harvester, 1986).
89. Donald Acheson, *AIDS* (London: RSM, 1988); R. J. Donaldson and L. J. Donaldson, *Essential Public Health Medicine* (Dordrecht: Kluwer, 1993); B. M. Davies and Tom Davies, *Community Health, Preventive Medicine and Social Services* (London: Baillière Tindall, 1993).

5

Social Medicine and Medical Sociology 1950–1970: The Testimony of a Partisan Participant

Margot Jefferys

Introduction

This paper is essentially about the relationships which developed between proponents of two emergent sub-disciplines – social medicine and medical sociology – in the UK academic scene from early in the 1950s until about 1970. It is based mainly on my recollection of events in which I was a participant, most often as a minor player rather than a leading actor. For most of the period I was a lecturer in social aspects of public health at the London School of Hygiene and Tropical Medicine. My experience in that particular location has inevitably coloured the opinions I express and the judgements I make.

I start with a description of the circumstances in the Department of Public Health at the London School of Hygiene and Tropical Medicine (hereafter LSHTM) when I joined it in the autumn of 1952. By circumstances I mean both its research and teaching interests. I follow by sketching with a broad brush the contemporary issues and approaches to their subject matter which characterized the main disciplines from which the two sub-disciplines sprang in the early 1950s. After that, I discuss some of the salient developments in the organizational growth of academic public health, social medicine and medical sociology during the 1950s and 1960s against a background of the external factors influencing those developments.

Throughout, the reader is asked to consider the influence of developments in the wider arena of health services and academia on the nature and quality of the relationships between public health (or social medicine) doctors and medical sociologists. Elsewhere, I have focused on the significance of the events of the 1950s and 1960s for the subsequent development of a Faculty of Community Medicine.[1]

Elsewhere too I have provided an autobiographical account of my personal involvement in the early years of identifying medical sociology as a field of academic study in the UK.[2] Here I draw on both those publications and on a short paper I contributed to a festschrift number of the journal *Public Health* in honour of Alwyn Smith in 1991.[3] There I considered the interdisciplinary relationships between medical sociologists and public health doctors in a more extended period.

Public Health Teaching and Research in the Early 1950s

When I joined the Public Health Department of the LSHTM in late 1952, I came into an establishment on the threshold of change. Its main function was to prepare qualified medical practitioners for the academic Diploma in Public Health, a statutory requirement for those who wished to become Medical Officers of Health in the elaborate local government structure of the United Kingdom. By 1953, however, a considerable proportion of the Department's diploma (DPH) students were from Third World, mainly Commonwealth countries.[4]

There were several assumptive bases for the DPH course, two of which are relevant here. The first was that the major threats to the public's health were from bacteria and viruses, and that they could be conquered primarily by strict control of the physical environment, by the imposition of mass prophylactic procedures such as vaccination, and by simple health education of the public. The last, according to the received wisdom of the time, should be directed particularly to working-class mothers who should be instructed in ways of preventing lethal infections and of sustaining infant growth by providing their offspring with better nutrition and following rudimentary personal hygiene measures.

The second assumption was that the measures needed to improve public health at local and national level had to be directed by doctors. Medical leadership over those who were to perform the various tasks dictated by such a wide public health programme was essential. Doctors were to be the strategists, determining the policy and ultimately responsible for the work done by those employed to carry out the various resulting tasks.

The result of these two assumptions was that the DPH postgraduate students were required to cover, if inevitably superficially, a wide range of subjects, in order to give credibility to their claim to be fit to exercise authority over the various non-medically qualified staff who carried out the wide range of public health functions in local government. A further consequence was that the Department had either to include some members of staff from disciplines other than medicine or to call in lecturers from outside to meet the needs generated by the syllabus.

The subjects taught, indeed, covered a wide range. They included elements of bacteriology and parasitology; but the main emphasis was on methods of environmental control to ensure clean water and food supplies, the disposal of waste products, and the creation and maintenance of minimum housing and public buildings standards. Immunization procedures were taught from the standpoint of the technology and its effectiveness. The DPH course also included an introduction to statistical methods and epidemiology.

Attention was also given to the problems of infant and childhood growth and deviations from normal health in order to prepare students to conduct or give guidance to those conducting medical and nursing surveillance in infant welfare and school health examinations.

In teaching all these subjects, the general assumption appeared to be that the UK experience would be appropriate preparation for those who were preparing to work anywhere else in the world. Even if they had no intention of working in British local government posts, students were expected to have a precise knowledge of British public health legislation and the legal duties of the UK's local authority Medical Officers of Health. More general education in administration or management method, or in those social sciences which had potentially something to contribute to the understanding of the role of social, cultural and economic factors in the determination of diversity in the health of different publics, had no place in the syllabus.

Signs of Change

By 1953, however, a slight breeze, rather than a stiff wind of change, had begun to blow through the corridors of the LSHTM and the Public Health Department in particular. The breeze was created by the appointment of John Brotherston to the Department as Reader in 1951.[5] An Edinburgh graduate in history before qualifying in medicine, he had studied at Johns Hopkins School of Public Health in Baltimore, USA. There he had been exposed to a much wider concept of the public health function than that which was still typically held by UK academic departments of public health. In particular, he had been excited by some Harvard social anthropologists who had stressed the cultural factors influencing both the nature of health problems in any society as well as the difficulties of changing health behaviours in developing societies which did not share beliefs in the efficacy of western-style medical practices.[6]

After Brotherston took up his appointment he got the willing if passive support of the Department head, Professor Sir James Mackintosh – one-time Medical Officer of Health for Glasgow – to introduce a number of innovative teaching methods. These included joint study groups with Health Visitors taking a tutor's course at the Royal College of Nursing. These undertook mini-research projects during the academic year and reported to the class as a whole at its end. Elective seminars for DPH students and postgraduate social anthropologists particularly interested in health and health care in African and Asian societies were also instituted at the London School of Economics and were led jointly by Professor Raymond Firth and myself.

It was Brotherston too who was responsible for persuading Mackintosh to appoint a social scientist (me) a post hitherto held by a medically qualified person. My main teaching responsibility was to broaden students' interests in the historical and contemporary social and economic contexts in which health and social welfare policies were formed and which lay behind the need for public health measures. Another of Brotherston's important contributions was to initiate a substantial research programme aimed at understanding the health and social effects of a large-scale re-housing scheme – the Oxhey study.[7] It was financed by a Rockefeller Foundation grant. The multi-disciplinary team engaged in it notably included a non-medically qualified statistician, Ann Cartwright,[8] fresh from a rigorous training in the Government Social Survey, and a social psychologist from the London School of Economics, Fred Martin.[9] Unfortunately for the LSHTM but not for health service research in general, these two followed John Brotherston to Scotland when he left to take up the Edinburgh University Chair of Social Medicine in 1956.

The gradual change in the assumptions made in the Public Health Department at the LSHTM about what future Medical Officers of Health required in the way of preparation for their role was also taking place in some of the other universities with a major commitment to postgraduate training in public health, and in particular in Edinburgh, Manchester and Belfast.[10] Elsewhere too, parallel changes were taking place. In particular, the Department of

Social Medicine at Birmingham University, led by Professor Tom McKeown, and the MRC Units devoted to elucidating the influence of social factors on specific aspects of health were breaking new ground and involving social scientists in their research.

Broadly speaking, the creation and work of these Units reflected the new approach to the role of medicine in both disease prevention and health promotion as well as in cure and comfort which had been sparked off by the ideas of John Ryle a decade earlier.[11] They also made use of sophisticated statistical methods to draw inferences about the causal complexities involved in the incidence or prevalence of disease and its consequences. Austin (Tony) Bradford Hill's influence in this area in retrospect can be seen as seminal.[12]

Given the new emphasis in all these departments and units on describing and explaining the wide social disparities in the distribution of disease, it was not surprising that some of their heads or directors should seek out social scientists to see what they could contribute to the understanding of their problems.

The Social Sciences in the 1950s

At this point, I propose to provide a broad picture of the intellectual preoccupations of mainstream sociologists and the organizational stage of development reached in the social sciences, and in sociology in particular, in British universities in the early 1950s. It is necessary to sketch such a picture in order to understand the nature of the approaches which were made to social scientists by social medicine exponents.

In the UK, academic departments of sociology were few in number. The most prestigious universities, Oxford and Cambridge, had steadfastly refused to establish one. The rejection in both instances was in part at least due to the hostility of other already established social science interests in these universities, namely economics and anthropology.[13] London, thanks to the existence of a constituent school, the London School of Economics (LSE), devoted entirely to the social sciences, had the premier department. It was still headed in the early 1950s by Morris Ginsberg, whose approach to his discipline was essentially philosophical.

A new, more empirically based approach to social structure was just beginning to make inroads there, thanks to the appointment of David Glass to a chair in the department;[14] but, in the early 1950s, little interest was shown by any mainstream sociologists in health status or health-related behaviour as social variables or in health services as social institutions, despite the concentration on social class as the major form of stratified societal division in the contemporary world.[15] The proponents of social medicine and of a new vision of the public health mission, however, did find a more favourable response from a rather peculiarly British brand of academics – who generally called themselves rather vaguely 'social scientists'. They had variously begun life as economists, economic historians or political scientists and had moved into academic departments which encouraged them to study issues associated with poverty and the means of alleviating it or modifying its concomitant results.

The most notable of this breed was Richard Titmuss, an autodidactic, degree-less actuarial insurance clerk. As a result of his formidable studies of infant mortality and a history of social policy during the Second World War years, he was appointed to a Chair of Social Policy and Administration at the LSE in 1952.[16]

The intellectual, essentially eclectic analysis of current socio-political trends typically made by this breed of social analysts and reformers represented a blend of Marxist and Fabian ideas. They were interested in the role of government, professions and voluntary agencies in changing public opinion and redistributing market-determined resource allocations. They were also committed to the view that the health of all was essential to the whole society and hence required social regulation and the planned control of services designed to deal with and prevent disease. They were, therefore, receptive to the suggestion that empirical enquiries, using quantitative survey methods, were necessary to help demonstrate the extent and nature of vulnerability and the need for treatment and cure which theoretically could be met at least in part by planned state provision. I believe that this position describes the stances taken by individuals like Richard Titmuss, who had already become a collaborator and close friend of Jerry Morris.

The Nucleus of 'Medical Sociologists'

Some of the social scientists who were actually drawn into the academic departments of public health or MRC units, and I count myself and Raymond Illsley among them, could be said to belong broadly to this mould of British social scientists. I had started life as an economic historian, done socio-economic research for the Ministry of Works in the immediate post-war years, and came under the influence of Barbara Wootton[17] during a short stint of work at Bedford College from 1950 to 1953. Raymond Illsley, a PPE Oxford graduate, was appointed to the MRC Unit in Social Obstetrics headed by Dugald Baird in Aberdeen, after some New

Town housing research in the late 1940s.[18]

Others came from the social anthropology stable. For example, prominent in the field were George Brown and Joe Loudon, both social anthropologists who joined the MRC Unit in Social Psychiatry at the Maudsley Institute of Psychiatry led by Aubrey Lewis;[19] Derek Allcorn, also a social anthropologist, and Tilda Goldberg, a psychiatric social worker, were taken on by Jerry Morris at the Social Medicine Research Unit, which moved during the mid-1950s from the Central Middlesex Hospital to the London Hospital Medical College.[20] Together, despite our disparate origins we began to be described collectively as medical sociologists, although, as far as I am aware none of us had had a primary academic qualification in sociology.

The Experience of the 1950s and 1960s

What happened to this somewhat spuriously labelled group of medical sociologists during the 1950s and 1960s? What kind of parts were we called upon to play in research and teaching? What kind of professional relationships did we make with those who had invited us in?

In 1955, on the initiative of Sir Harold Himsworth, its secretary, the MRC showed itself willing to consider making a more substantial investment in social research relevant to health and health service provision. It called a meeting in that year to which it invited an array of prominent epidemiologists and other medically qualified scientists with interests in health care policy, several leading professors of social anthropology, and the few social scientists already employed in MRC Units and academic departments of public health or social medicine.[21]

From the standpoint of those of us who wanted to see a greater commitment on the part of the MRC and increasing job opportunities within academic departments in the medical faculties, the meeting was a disaster. Its proceedings were dominated by Max Gluckman of Manchester and Meyer Fortes of Cambridge, neither of whom were particularly interested in securing research resources for themselves or their students from the Council. Raymond Firth, on the other hand, was, and he was bitterly disappointed by the stance adopted by his two anthropology colleagues. They gave a display of intellectual arrogance by subjecting the distinguished epidemiologists to didactic lectures suitable for undergraduate beginners on anthropological concepts and methods. At the same time they refused to enter into any kind of meaningful discourse on issues which were of genuine concern to the epidemiologists such as the nature of the inferences made in small-scale, individually conducted observational studies typical of many undertaken by social anthropologists at the time. There is little doubt that the meeting helped to reinforce the view held by many medically qualified epidemiologists that social scientists, whatever the protestations of their exponents, had little to offer serious medical researchers.

Indeed, until the mid-1960s, the climate in British academia remained generally unfavourable to the development of any substantial sociologically oriented research in the health field. There were, however, a number of encouraging signs. The newly founded Society for Social Medicine decided to open its membership to non-medically qualified scientists on roughly the same terms as to medically qualified ones.[22] John Brotherston, at the LSHTM, took the initiative in founding a multi-disciplinary discussion group – the Keppel Club – which met monthly to exchange views on broad health policy issues, and social scientists from both within and outside the medical schools became members.[23] The MRC did not lose faith in the social scientists already in its employ and continued to facilitate meetings of those working in different units and public health departments. This helped to give us a sense of identity, and, simultaneously, we began to receive some recognition from colleagues for our contribution to research.

All the same, most of us experienced the reluctance on the part of medically qualified co-workers adequately to acknowledge our contribution by putting our names as joint authors, let alone as main authors, on papers submitted to medical journals.[24] More seriously, we found our path to senior posts within medically led institutions barred, while less meritorious also-rans with medical qualifications climbed effortlessly up the academic ladder. It was only too often the latter who had the authority to set the research agendas in which they expected social scientists to play a subordinate role.

Given the lack of autonomy, the poor promotion prospects, the job insecurity for most of those recruited to undertake fieldwork on research projects designed by others, not to speak of the hostility or indifference with which dragooned medical students treated those who tried to lecture to them, it was not surprising that most of those who came into medically led departments with some enthusiasm left after a year or two. The most able of them, resentful of what they considered demeaning treatment received from the medical establishment, drifted back, often with reluctance, to mainstream social science departments or into research in other fields where they could secure greater psychic rewards and firmer career prospects.

My personal experience during the mid-1960s exemplifies the dilemma faced by some of us who had made a whole-hearted commitment to research in the health field. After a two-month tour of schools and departments of public health in the USA in 1963, where I saw social scientists accorded much more recognition and responsibility than was the case in the UK,[25] I tried to get the LSHTM to establish a medical sociology unit independent of the Public Health Department. Its purpose would be to provide training posts for doctoral and post-doctoral students who wished to work on issues related to health and health services. The reputation of the Public Health Department at that point in time, however, was at a deservedly low ebb, thanks to weak – one might almost say non-existent – intellectual leadership. I hoped that an independent unit with two or three career posts for lecturer-researchers and a postgraduate studentship programme would encourage able social science students to enter a field which I had found rewarding and wished to see further developed.

I was unsuccessful in my bid, and, as a consequence and with some reluctance, left in 1965 to accept a Readership in the Sociology Department at Bedford College which also carried the title of Director of a newly formed Social Research Unit. I was joined there in 1969 by George Brown who had been similarly discouraged about the possibility of pursuing the research which he felt was feasible and necessary in the MRC's Social Psychiatry Research Unit at the Institute of Psychiatry.[26] By 1970 we both had personal chairs and had started a postgraduate master's degree course in the sociology of medicine, assisted initially by the Nuffield Foundation.[27] It continues today and has turned out a stream of people, many of whom went on to obtain doctorates and posts at senior levels in medically led academic departments, and MRC and health authority research units.[28]

Another Contemporary Controversy

It was perhaps the widespread perception that social scientists working from within a medical faculty appeared not to be able to make a truly independent contribution to the education of future doctors or to research on health or health service matters that led, in the late 1960s, to the recommendation made by the Royal Commission on Medical Education on the teaching of medical sociology in the medical curriculum.[29] It was to the effect that the contribution of sociological theory and practice to basic medical education should be made by sociologists employed by the universities' mainstream sociology departments and not by those working in medical faculties. A similar proposal was made for the teaching of medical psychology.

In support of the recommendation it was argued that the most gifted behavioural scientists were unlikely to opt to work within medical faculties for a variety of reasons. First, for example, they would not have the opportunity to interact with their own true peers from whom they might soon be cut off, thus losing contact with advanced thinking in their parent discipline. Secondly, they would not have the opportunity to teach students of their own discipline. 'Service' teaching of medical students could not, in itself, be intellectually stimulating. Thirdly, medical scientists and clinicians were unlikely to treat social scientists as professional equals unless they had an equivalent academic status to their own.

These were powerful arguments, but I was opposed to them at the time and continue to feel that they were wrong.[30] I argued that, if the subject was to be both well taught and credible to medical students, those who taught it had to be seen to be as much immersed in the medical enterprise as the other teachers providing the basic knowledge required by all medical graduates or those specializing in specific fields of public health.[31]

Of course, since then, time has marched on. Most medical faculties in Britain now employ social scientists directly. They are attached to one or other department (not necessarily departments of social or community or public health medicine) and are expected to fulfil the GMC's recommended guidelines that all medical students should be introduced to some of those elements of the discipline of greatest relevance to the understanding of medical practice. Although some medical faculties have failed to make full-time appointments, at the time of writing they all appear to use the services of social scientists who are employed in one or other medical department rather than those employed in university departments of sociology. Moreover, sociologists no longer are confined to the most junior posts within the faculty. Several sociologists have personal chairs and several readerships. Some have doctorates awarded within the medical faculty. At the LSHTM, social scientists are present in considerably greater numbers than they were in the 1960s.

In other words there has been a breakthrough which reflects at least an increasing openness on the part of medical educators and researchers to respond to outside pressures. These pressures require that doctors be better equipped with knowledge of the social context within which they live and work and with empathy for patients with cultural assumptions different from their own.[32]

The Matrimonial Imagery

Returning in my concluding comments to the relationships between the sub-disciplines of social medicine and medical sociology in the 1950s and 1960s, I propose to use the metaphor of courtship and marriage to describe them. It was used wittily by Fred Martin, who died tragically young, in a talk he gave in 1976 during a seminar organized by Roy Acheson. Medicine and sociology were then [he was referring to the 1960s] being joined, smiling, in holy wedlock – but has it proved to be holy wedlock or wholly deadlock? It is obvious in retrospect that marital expectations were fallacious from the beginning: no-one questioned that medicine was the male partner, kindly, benevolent, but a bit of a chauvinist. However, it turned out that the bride was a dedicated member of the women's liberation movement, and intended to spend her time in marriage, not performing her duties along the lines laid down by her partner, but in proclaiming the autonomy of sociology and denouncing medical domination.[33]

Martin concluded then that what had been accomplished thus far at an interdisciplinary level had fallen far short of legitimate expectations. I agree in the main with his conclusion and accept that his metaphor expressed delightfully and truthfully some of the elements which helped to sour the relationship. In fact, I propose to extend the metaphor and use its imagery to provide more insight into the relationship and why it was so often an uneasy one.

First, we should note that the betrothal was not looked upon with much favour by either of the couple's parents. On the groom's side, the parents – mainstream clinical medicine – to whom the groom could not help but be nostalgically attached, had never had much affection for the public health/social medicine espoused by their wayward offspring. Nor had they approved the company that that offspring had kept in local government or the interest shown in matters other than clinical medicine. Now that offspring was making the even more outrageous proposal to bring into the parental home a very low-status bedfellow, a possible cuckoo in the nest. They could not but disapprove. The bride, perhaps preoccupied with the problems which she was encountering from her own parents, may have been insufficiently sensitive to those faced by her intended spouse.

On the bride's side too there was plenty of parental disapproval of the match. Sociology departments were seeking to establish their *bona fides* within academia and did not want their few cherished offspring to flirt with members of other departments, and particularly not with medicine which, while powerful within the academic hierarchy, sociologists were apt to hold in contempt as a-intellectual if not anti-intellectual. Those of their offspring who were willing to consort with the medical profession could be accused of prostitution.

Siblings of both groom and bride, that is, other developing specialities, were also not over-enthusiastic. If the relationship thrived it could lead to a larger share of their family's scarce resources going to the couple at the expense of all those who were leading virtuous lives with no untoward liaisons.

Given these signs of, to say the least, parental ambivalence, it was not surprising to find some hesitations on the part of one or both parties to the association. Furthermore, doubts increased when it became clear, after early honeymoon euphoria, that both parties had not been altogether clear about their partner's intellectual credentials, objectives, underlying beliefs and motivations. Epidemiologists, who had already established good relations with statisticians to whom they could usually put straightforward questions, found that sociologists were often not merely innumerate but, perhaps as a result, dismissive of their concerns with precise measurement and quantification. Sociologists, on the other hand, were irritated by the epidemiologists' tendency to restrict data collection to only those questions which they considered would throw light on already formulated hypotheses.

The use of the matrimonial metaphor is, I believe, helpful in explaining why the social medicine–medical sociology relationship, despite its intrinsically sensible promise, was not an easy one in the 1950s and 1960s and still faces tensions today.

It would not be correct, however, to suggest that the experience of collaboration which took place during those decades was a failure. New ground was broken: both disciplines learned enough from each other to alter the terms of their own discourse and, ultimately, to influence together the more general discourse relating to many aspects of the global health and health care enterprise.

Acknowledgements

Many friends and colleagues have helped refresh my memory and directed me to sources which have either confirmed my recollections or made me, in some way, modify the assertions in the initial oral presentation of the paper. I would like to thank, in particular, Joyce

Allcorn, George Brown, Ann Cartwright, Tilda Goldberg, Raymond Illsley, Ann Oakley and Michael Shepherd.

Editor's note: Margot Jeffreys wishes to point out that this essay was written as a personal reflection of events and completed before the publication of some recent studies which are especially relevant to her subject, such as the history of the Faculty of Community Medicine, authored by Michael Warren.*

*Michael Warren, *The Genesis of the Faculty of Community Medicine, Now the Faculty of Public Health Medicine* (Kent: Centre for Health Service Studies, the University of Kent, 1997).

Notes

1. Jefferys, M., 'The Transition from Public Health to Community Medicine: The Evolution and Execution of a Policy for Occupational Transformation', *Bulletin of the Society for the Social History of Medicine*, 39 (1986), 47–63.
2. Jefferys, M., 'Serendipity: an Autobiographical Account of the Career of a Medical Sociologist in Britain,' in R. H. Elling and M. Sokolowska (eds), *Medical Sociologists at Work* (New Brunswick, N.J.: Transactions Press,1978), 135–61.
3. Jefferys, M., 'Medical Sociology and Public Health:Inter-disciplinary Relationships, 1950–90,' *Public Health*, 109 (1991), 15–21.
4. The Annual Reports of the London School of Hygiene and Tropical Medicine do not give the nationalities of the DPH students separately from those of all students. One-third of the latter were from Great Britain, another third from Third World Commonwealth countries.
5. John Brotherston, 1915–85, joined the LSHTM 1950. Promoted to Readership in 1951. Chair of Public Health & Social Medicine Edinburgh University 1955–64. Chief Medical Officer Scotland 1964–77. Returned to Edinburgh Chair 1977. Obituary by George Godber, *BMJ* , 290 (1985), 1670.
6. Benjamin Paul, editor of *Health, Culture & Community: Case Studies of Public Health Reactions to Health Programs* (New York: Russell Sage, 1955), was at Harvard School of Public Health when Brotherston was in the USA. Other social anthropologists who influenced him were Edward G. Spicer, *Human Problems in Technological Change* (New York: Russell Sage, 1952) and Lyle Saunders, *Cultural Difference and Medical Care* (New York: Russell Sage,1954).
7. Jefferys, M., 'Londoners in Hertfordshire,' in R. Glass and J. Westergaard (eds), *London: Aspects of Change* (London: MacGibbon & Kee, 1964), 207–55, gives a general description of the

study, and a list of papers reporting the results of the study.

8. Ann Cartwright, 1925–, ultimately founded and directed the Institute for Social Studies in Medical Care 1970–93. She was the author (sole or joint) of a voluminous output of books and papers relating to various aspects of medical care and survey methods. Her c.v. and copies of her publications are available in the Contemporary Archive of the Wellcome Institute's History of Medicine, London.
9. Fred Martin, 1923–87, coauthored with Jean Floud and A. H. Halsey *Social Class and Educational Opportunity* (London: Routledge & Kegan Paul, 1956). He joined Brotherston as a lecturer in the Department of Social Medicine in 1956. He left Edinburgh in 1967 to become Assistant Director of Research & Intelligence at the Greater London Council and then Director of Social Research & Policy, before returning to Scotland in 1973 as Professor of Social Administration in the University of Glasgow, unfortunately dying while still in office.
10. Crew, F. A. E., 1886–1973, was Brotherston's predecessor in Edinburgh. Fraser Brockington, 1903–, was making important changes to the Manchester teaching of public health. A talented group in Queen's, Belfast, which included John Pemberton, 1912–, Maurice Backett, 1916–, Peter Froggart, 1928–, and Eric Cheeseman, 1912–87 (a medical statistician), was also breaking new ground in teaching and research.
11. John Ryle, 1889–1950. Michael Shepherd gives a brief account of his life and work in the Preface (xi–xix) to the reprint of *The Natural History of Disease* published by the Keynes Press for the British Medical Association in 1988.
12. Austin (Tony) Bradford Hill, 1900–91. The journal *Statistics in Medicine*, (1) (2) (1982), was a *festschrift* issue in his honour containing essays by 13 epidemiologists and statisticians including Richard Doll.
13. Bulmer, M. in Bulmer, M. (ed.), *Essays on the History of British Sociological Research* (Cambridge: Cambridge University Press, 1985), 25–8. In the same volume, Halsey, A. H. (151–64) and Shils, E. (165–78) also discuss the reasons for the failure to develop independent departments of sociology at Oxford and Cambridge.
14. David Glass, 1911–78. His influence on social demography in the immediate post-war period resulted largely from his involvement in the Population Investigation Committee's enquiries, undertaken for the Royal Commission on Population. Research Papers 1–6 (London: HMSO, 1949–54), and *Report,* Cmd. 7695 (London: HMSO, 1949).
15. Glass, D. V. (ed.), *Social Mobility in Britain* (London: Routledge &

Kegan Paul, 1954). See Willmott, P., 'The Institute of Community Studies', in M. Bulmer (ed.), *Essays on the History of British Sociological Research* (Cambridge: Cambridge University Press, 1985), 137–50, for a brief history of the Institute of Community Studies (founded 1953–4) and of the publications of its major research workers, Michael Young, Peter Townsend, Peter Marris and Peter Willmott. In my view, Young's outstanding contribution, in a life studded with major contributions to social thought and social action, was *The Rise of the Meritocracy* (London: Thames & Hudson, 1962). As far as I am aware he was the first person to coin the term 'meritocracy'.

16. Titmuss, Richard M., 1907–73. Margaret Gowing wrote an appreciation in *The Proceedings of the British Academy*, Vol. LXI (1975). Abel-Smith, B. and Titmuss, K. (eds), *The Philosophy of Welfare. Selected Writings of Richard Titmuss* (1987), contains both an appreciation and a bibliography.
17. One of the most distinguished radical thinkers of the century was Barbara Wootton,1897–1988. She left her mark in a number of books which included *Social Science and Social Pathology* (London: Allen & Unwin, 1959). Her autobiography, *A World I Never Made,* was published in 1967.
18. Dugald Baird, 1899–1986. Regius Professor of Midwifery in the University of Aberdeen since 1937, he started recruiting dietitians, sociologists, psychologists and statisticians to his department in 1948, and the MRC made him Honorary Director of the Obstetric Research Unit in Aberdeen in 1955, a post he held until he retired in 1965. The Unit was then transformed into the Medical Sociology Research Unit whose first director was Raymond Illsley.
19. Aubrey Lewis, 1900–75. See an appreciation by Michael Shepherd, 'From Social Medicine to Social Psychiatry: The achievement of Sir Aubrey Lewis', *Psychological Medicine* (10) (1980), 211–18. For G. W. Brown see reference 26 below.
20. J. N. Morris, 1910–. Director of the Social Medicine Research Unit 1948–74. Best known for his book *The Uses of Epidemiology,* first published in 1957 and subsequently republished three times. Several sociologists worked in the SMRU, including Derek Allcorn, 1927–86, a social anthropologist, who, after completing a Manchester Ph.D. thesis on young men, joined Morris's Unit in London from 1955 to 1958 and then Dugald Baird's in Aberdeen until 1960. Tilda Goldberg, 1912–, a psychiatric social worker by training, also had an important role in the MRC Social Medicine Unit. She published her study of young men with peptic ulcers in

1958 under the title *Family Influences and Psychosomatic Illness* (London: Tavistock). She was also the joint author with S. I. Morrison of a seminal paper, 'Schizophrenia & Social Class', *Brit J of Psychiatry,* 109 (1963), 785–802.

21. The meeting was held in 1956. The academic departments of social sciences were represented by professors of social anthropology rather than of sociology or social administration. Three men predominated. They were Max Gluckman of Manchester,1911–75, Meyer Fortes of Cambridge,1906–83, and Raymond Firth, London School of Economics, 1901–.
22. The early papers are held in the Wellcome Medical Archives (SA/SSM/A1,2 & 3). Early correspondence of the founders suggests that the chief concern was to exclude those Medical Officers of Health who were not themselves engaged in research, rather than those without medical qualifications who were active in academic departments and research units.
23. Fry, J., 'The Keppel Club (1952–74): lessons from the past for the future', *BMJ,* 303 (1991), 1596–8, gives an account of its formation and early meetings and includes a list of its members during the 1950s.
24. In 1965, the *Lancet* reordered the names on a paper submitted to them to give precedence to my two medical collaborators, although I was the main author. The editor subsequently apologized when we informed him that we would not publish if the names were not given in their original order. [M. Jefferys, S. Gauvain and O. Guleson, 'Comparison of Men and Women in Medical Training', *Lancet,* i (1965), 1361–3.]
25. I was a visiting WHO Fellow from March to June 1963 and presented a report of my visit to US schools of public health and departments of medical sociology to both the WHO sponsors and my department head at the LSHTM. I can find no trace of it among my personal papers.
26. George Brown, 1930–. Since 1980 has been honorary Professor of Sociology, University of London and on the External Staff of the MRC. Initially supported by a grant from the SSRC, he has subsequently received extensive support from the MRC and various American foundations for his studies of the effect of social structural and behavioural factors on various forms of illness including depression, heart conditions and cancer. His major publications include 'Social Factors Influencing Length of Hospital Stay of Schizophrenic Patients', *BMJ* (2) (1959), 1300–4; with J. K. Wing, *Institutionalism and Schizophrenia* (Cambridge: Cambridge

University Press, 1970); with T. O. Harris, *Social Origins of Depression: A Study of Psychiatric Disorder in Women* (London: Tavistock, 1978).

27. The Nuffield Foundation provided Bedford College with a three-year grant in 1969 to employ an assistant lecturer, on the understanding that the College itself would continue to fund the post if the projected one-year M.Sc. course in Sociology as Applied to Medicine attracted sufficient good graduates. It did, and still runs today under the direction of Professor Mike Bury.
28. One of the earliest M.Sc. students was Sally McIntyre, at present Director of the MRC Medical Sociology Research Unit at Glasgow University. Many other students are now engaged in teaching and/or research in social science and medical academic departments.
29. Royal Commission on Medical Education, 1965–8 (the *Todd Report*) (London: HMSO, 1969), Cmnd 3569, paras 257–9.
30. My views were expressed in 'Sociology and Medicine: Separation or Symbiosis', *Lancet*, i (1969), 1111–16.
31. I further expressed my views on the role of medical sociology in medical education in 'Does Medicine Need Sociology?' in D. Tuckett and J. M. Kaufert (eds), *Basic Readings in Medical Sociology* (London: Tavistock, 1978), and in 'Sociology and Medical Education in Britain: A Sociologic Analysis of their Relationship,' *International Journal of Health Services* (4) (1974), 549–63.
32. A group of sociology lecturers in London medical schools produced a textbook in 1980 which was revised in a third edition in 1991 – evidence of the increasing acceptance of the subject as a legitimate part of the medical curriculum. G. Scambler (ed.), *Sociology as Applied to Medicine* (London: Baillière's Concise Medical Textbook, 3rd edition, 1991).
33. Martin, F. M., 'Comments on Sociology and Community Medicine,' in R. M. Acheson and L. Aird (eds), *Seminars in Community Medicine.* Vol. 1. *Sociology* (London: Oxford University Press, 1976), 17.

6

The Dilemma of Social Pathology

Uta Gerhardt

Introduction

Social pathology was originally introduced in the USA as an approach to the analysis of social problems; it focused on illness as one among many aspects of individual or social disintegration. Through the work of the Chicago School of Sociology, if indirectly, social pathology became the stepping-stone for the sociology of illness that conceptualized the problems of social definition and dominance. In the 1970s, this approach was introduced in Britain as a framework for understanding the dynamics of doctor–patient encounters. Its aim was to show that the patient harboured a view of illness that was equal to, if not independent of, that of the doctor. Taking the side of the patient in this manner was also a political stance epitomizing two critical attitudes *vis-à-vis* medicine. One was directed against the so-called medical model inasmuch as it represented patient-aversive medical care. The other was directed against medicine's as well as medical sociology's analytical focus on illness rather than health. The rationale for the latter criticism was that sociology as a practical discipline wanted to contribute to an understanding of health as a positive goal for humankind rather than illness as a negative state that was to be avoided. From this vantage point, *suffering* constituted the human condition whose overcoming had to be a foremost goal of sociological work. This conception of sociology's task made the International Sociological Association's Research Committee No. 15 change its name from 'Sociology of Medicine' into 'Sociology of Health' in 1986.

In order to understand the particular perspectives taken by British medical sociology as of the 1970s, it is necessary to trace the history of the approach in the USA from its early period, the 1920s, to its peak period in the 1960s. Such historical account shows how the social pathology perspective in medical sociology emerged from the more general social-problems approach taken by social pathologists since the early twentieth century.

The framework of social pathology, as it has developed, contains two sides of a dilemma. One side is related to methods. Most social pathology research claims to use a naturalistic approach geared at social problems as the 'natural history' or experienced phenomenon. The dilemma concerns the objectivity claim of scientific knowledge. The other side of the dilemma is related to theory. Most social pathology writings conceptualize illness as a social or cultural construction. The dilemma concerns the meaning of illness when society is deemed all-pervasive but the individual's freedom is endorsed wholeheartedly.

This chapter has three parts and a concluding section. First, some of the history of the analysis of social pathology in American sociology is reconstructed. Second, the contribution of British medical sociology is highlighted, focusing on the 1970s. Third, the dilemma of sociological thought that is based on the social pathology framework is outlined. The concluding part looks beneath and beyond the dilemma.

The Development of the Social Pathology Framework

Between 1925 and 1951, six books were published in the USA under the same title, *Social Pathology* (Queen and Mann, 1925; Mangold, 1932/4; Gillin, 1933/39/46; Queen and Gruener, 1940; Brown, 1942; Lemert, 1951). The earliest, by Stuart Queen and Delbert Mann, outlined an array of social problems that signified social pathology. They were, among others, blindness, deafness, drug addiction, alcoholism, suicide, divorce, illegitimacy, prostitution, old age, homelessness, and mental breakdown or deficiency. These areas of non-integration into society were analysed under two perspectives. One was that individuals who came under those labels did not fit into society and had to be submitted to corrective measures such as punishment or treatment. The other was that social problems suggested social disintegration; this meant that poverty, parental neglect or other unfavourable conditions of life during socialization could make it practically impossible for an adolescent to fit into society. Therefore, social reform as a community effort had to counteract social pathology, supplementing social work and education as an individual effort. The idea was that through such double policy society should be made an adequate life-world for all citizens. The idea remained the book's message in its second much-revised edition published in the early period of the Second World War (Queen and Gruener, 1940). Its new subtitle was *Obstacles to Social Participation.*

Before he published a monograph devoted to *Social Pathology* (1933, revised in 1939, and again in 1946), John Gillin made social pathology one of four major areas of sociological thought in his *Outlines of Sociology* (3rd revised edition, 1930). Together with the three topics of social evolution, socialization and collectivities, and 'social ideals and social control' which included government as well as education, social pathology represented a primary field of sociological interest. He defined 'the nature of social pathology' as follows:

> Social pathology refers to the maladjustments in social relationships ... The term ... may be used to denote the social conditions which result (1) from failure of individuals so to adjust themselves to social life that they function as independent, self-supporting members of society, who contribute their fair share to its stability and progressive development, and (2) from the lack of adjustment of social structure, including ways of doing things and institutions, to the development of social personality. Pathological conditions in society may result from (1) natural lack of ability in individuals to keep pace with the changing ideals and institutions of society, or (2) from the failure of society to keep pace in its functional machinery with the changing conditions in the world in which it lives. (Gillin and Blackmar, 1930: 527)

Although entire societies might be or become pathological, Gillin stated, the more usual situation was that a 'particular class of people within a social group or ... a defective function of government' (*ibid.*: 539) caused the 'pathology of education' leading to insufficient learning, inadequate attitudes toward information, or lack of a sense of responsibility as citizen, and also 'pathology in industry' (e.g. child labour, replacement of men by machines causing mass unemployment) or in the economy (where the Great Depression prevailed into the 1930s). Among the three topics discussed in detail – in addition to poverty and crime – was that of 'social degeneration.' By this Gillin referred to alcoholism and immorality (sexual abuse, prostitution, etc.) undermining society's 'close-knit coordination and orderly functioning which is necessary for social progress' (*ibid.*: 629), as well as 'hereditary influences' (e.g. family disposition for mental retardation) and 'eugenics' ('the study of eugenics helps us to so direct social activity that better racial character may be developed and utilized' (*ibid.*: 632)); this led to his definition of 'social degeneration' as breakdown or deterioration of the 'effective coordination of individuals and groups' (*ibid.*: 633). In this context, Gillin mentioned illness as follows:

> The influence of disease from social groupings, unsanitory conditions, improper employment of men, women, and children, enforced idleness through the shifting of industrial life, and conditions which produce a high death rate, all have a decided effect in producing social degeneration. (*ibid.*)

In the early 1940s, Richard Fuller in two influential articles questioned the assumptions of *progressivism* in the earlier approach. Outlining a framework for explaining and teaching social problems (Fuller, 1940a; Fuller and Myers, 1941), he clarified that what figured as social pathology was predominantly determined by social factors of two kinds. On the one hand, progress of knowledge in medicine and other sciences made previously uncontrollable problems manageable. On the other hand, what figured as a social problem was defined by public opinion rendering certain deviations from normality intolerable. Fuller and Myers wrote:

> If the people are not problem-conscious, they will not behave as if there were any problem. They will not debate the condition as a problem nor will they organize to do anything about it. Social problems are what people think they are. (Fuller and Myers, 1941: 25)

Distinguishing between *physical* problems such as earthquakes, or epidemics prior to modern medicine, *ameliorative* problems such as murder or mental illness, and *moral* problems such as divorce, race prejudice, or war, Fuller stressed two points. First, when a problem was defined as moral, its identification as pathological depended on value standards that could be questioned by others who tolerated or benefited from the problem – epitomized by child labour or racial hatred. That is to say:

> Race prejudice in many sections of our country does not disturb many individuals at all. We can take a point here from Fascist persecution of the Jews. Race prejudice is defended by totalitarian authorities as a natural phenomenon – essential to the survival of the 'pure' racial strains. Even less need be said as to the absence of any clear national or world consensus which defines war as something wrong and in need of eradication at all costs. (*ibid.*: 31)

Second, the three classificatory groups were *relative* inasmuch as particular problems could 'move' from one to the other: 'When problems now classed as moral come to have wide disapproval throughout our culture as conditions which must in every instance be done away with, they will become essentially problems of solution rather than agreement on basic values and will be dealt with as ameliorative problems' (*ibid.*: 31).

The gist of the argument was that essentially no difference existed between normal and pathological issues except that social values interfered, rendering some problems moral and some ameliorative.

Such *relativism* was considered scientific since it overcame the moralistic undertone of sociology's previous analysis of social pathology. Fuller insisted that normal and pathological phenomena were similar social processes although evaluated differently; he found that social problems have a *natural history*, that is, a structure of a patterned sequence of stages, which likens them to any other field of sociological enquiry (Fuller, 1940b).

To overcome the dichotomy between the normal and the pathological, and to acknowledge the relativity of these classifications, became the novel focus of social pathology textbooks.

The first after Fuller's articles was Lawrence Guy Brown's *Social Pathology* (1942). It retained some of the traditional approach by focusing on *Personal and Social Disorganization* (its subtitle) but it incorporated the new view by not only stressing the relativity issue but also proposing a solution to its vicissitudes – scientific research. The book devoted three of its four parts to personal disorganization, and one to social disorganization. Under the label of personal disorganization fell speech disorders, sex pathologies, pathological eating or drinking, drug addiction, disorders of emotion, physical ill-health, mental ill-health, mental deficiency, suicide, and also psychopathic personality, and delinquents and criminals. Under social disorganization, among other topics, fell institutional misdevelopments in the economy, education, the family, the law, the press, religion, science, or the political sphere, and also war and 'social-psychological epidemics.' The latter referred to fascism under the perspective taken by psychiatry, namely, the analysis and criticism of mass-man (Strecker, 1940) particularly in the contemporary society: 'Just now, social-psychological epidemics of an abnormal nature seem to be the main form of social disorganization, involving the entire world' (Brown, 1942: 549). The pathology of fascist leadership, to be sure, was emphasized in no uncertain terms: 'A paranoid personality, with leadership aspirations, thrives in a sick society or in a society that believes itself discriminated against by some other group' (*ibid.*: 551).

Brown acknowledged the relativity perspective by placing social disorganization in a unified, albeit two-pronged, conceptual framework. 'Normal attitudes may be achieved in war and be expressed in a program of peace .... War does not have its meaning apart from economic, cultural, and political factors. The disorganized areas of a city have no meaning apart from the organized regions,' he wrote.

At this point, science entered the scene and broke up the impasse of relativism. 'The social scientist studies all behavior with the same procedure for both normal and abnormal activities. His approach and his attitudes are the same for data defined as social disorganization as they are for data regarded as social organization' (*ibid.*: 365). The scientific attitude, therefore, was to contribute toward the integration of the abnormal into society by acknowledging that between the normal and the deviant was a thin and often blurred line of distinction. The individual, then, comprised 'varying degrees of normality and abnormality.' Brown stated:

> Both normal and abnormal behavior are manifestations of human nature. This fact places the normal and the abnormal in the same broad category and makes them, in general, the same type of phenomenon; it also makes it possible to establish unifying principles that will apply to all social phenomena. Furthermore, the research student or the treatment specialist will never find a single situation where the abnormal is isolated from the normal. There are not two classes of people in society, the normal and the abnormal, but persons with varying degrees of normality and abnormality (*ibid.*: 57)

This solution to the relativity problem was taken up by Edwin Lemert's *Social Pathology*, published in 1951. It was the last book with this title and also the only one written after the Second World War. It drew on its predecessors in two obvious ways. First, Lemert followed the earlier approaches in that he defined social pathology as social problems, and, second, he assumed that to analyse normal and pathological phenomena using the same conceptual approach was scientific and also politically correct inasmuch as it carried a pro-democracy, anti-discriminatory political message.

Lemert wrote his book in order to provide a solution to what he perceived as the unsolved methodological problem of sociology, namely, how personal and social disorganization were related to each other (Lemert, 1951: 13). He referred to Fuller's ideas of relativity and natural history but avowed that he took a different path out of the muddle of moralistic and positivist previous analysis. He coined the term 'sociopathic behaviour' for the subject area of his perspective on social pathology. In substantive terms, it focused on seven areas discussed in most previous literature on social pathology – blindness, speech disorders, political extremism, prostitution, crime, alcoholism, and mental disorder. However, he addressed the dynamics of sociopathic behaviour while he realized that the social problem was different from the experience of the person who acquired the problematic behaviour or identity. Distinguishing between deviance and deviants, he saw a two-sided phenomenon; in effect, his chapters were entitled 'Blindness and the Blind,' 'Radicalism and Radicals,' 'Drunkenness and the Chronic Alcoholic,' etc. Through such double focus, he wanted to clarify that the relationship between motivation and action, personality and behaviour was the obverse of what the traditional perspective on social pathology had taken for granted. His conceptual model of the social process of becoming deviant was that sociopathic behaviour emerged through a three-stage process of symbolic interaction. It consisted of primary deviation (accidental deviance, even unusual behaviour or experiences), societal reaction (others' definition of the character of the behaviour and the value of the person whose behaviour deviated from usual expectations or standards once or more frequently), and sociopathic individuation (reaction of the person to the societal reaction, amounting to self-categorization in the terms used by significant others involved in the societal reaction, leading to subsequent development by the person or self of the respective attributed identity). Lemert insisted that motivation in the person did not bring about the sociopathic behaviour but, in contrast, was its consequence. This meant that a person perceived by others as a deviant developed the motivation and self befitting the deviant. In this vein, he said, sociopathic behaviour was frequently produced by categorization routines in treatment institutions. Whereas the latter were meant to re-integrate deviants into mainstream society, their function, however, was to alienate them further from it. Addressing the 'symbolic consequences of control,' he warned of iatrogenic effects of inadvertent labelling procedures in corrective or therapeutic agencies. He wrote:

> Among the unanticipated consequences of therapy, treatment, and administrative manipulations, none are more important than those

> which are symbolic in nature. More and more we are coming to realize that the actual symbolic impact of a control or therapeutic experience often is a far cry from what has been intended .... Court hearings, home investigations by social workers, arrests, clinical visits, segregation within the school system and other formal dispositions of deviants under the aegis of public welfare or public protection in many instances are cause for dramatic redefinitions of the self and role of deviants. (*ibid.*: 70–1)

The political message of Lemert's view of social pathology became obvious in the 1960s. Howard Becker, in *Outsiders* (1963), emphasized that deviant behaviour, as he phrased it, was 'behaviour that people so label' (Becker, 1963: 9) rather than action propelled by motivation originating in personal disorder or deficit. In particular, deviants were not people who were inferior to those who were normals but 'the deviant is one to whom that label has successfully been applied' (*ibid.*). That is, the person who was stigmatized as a drug addict, homosexual or mental patient was one to whom others had successfully applied the respective negative categories irrespective of whether or not they were justified or whether others who were not labelled might also engage in the stigmatizable behaviour.

In a similar vein, as Erving Goffman argued in *Asylums* (1961), whereas patients in mental hospitals usually had psychiatric symptoms, so did many among society's normals who were not hospitalized. He stated:

> The society's official view is that inmates of mental hospitals are there primarily because they are suffering from mental illness. However, in the degree that the 'mentally ill' outside hospital numerically approach or surpass those inside hospitals, one could say that mental patients distinctively suffer not from mental illness, but from contingencies. (Goffman, 1961: 135)

Whereas the analytical approach with which deviants were to be studied was the same for the normal and the pathological, the finding was that separate worlds existed for those who fully participated in society and those who were excluded from participation through stigmatization and subsequent discrimination. In *Stigma* (1963), Goffman argued that the blind, deaf, physically or mentally handicapped, etc. were discontinued in their previous personal as well as social identities, thus losing their original ego identity, and then were reconstituted as deviants with an identity of stigma that could nevertheless render them acceptable as second-class citizens to others. A similar process, although from birth or as early as school age, applied to Jews, Blacks, Japanese in the USA, etc. He said about the 'stigmatized individual's' fate and plight:

> He is encouraged to have distaste for those of his fellows who, without actually making a secret of their stigma, engage in careful covering, being very careful to show that in spite of appearances they are very sane, very generous, very sober, very masculine, very capable of hard physical labour and taxing sports, in short, that they are Gentlemen deviants, nice persons like ourselves in spite of the reputation of their kind. It should be plain that these advocated codes of conduct provide the stigmatized individual not merely with a platform and a politics, and not merely with instruction as to how to treat others, but with recipes for an appropriate attitude regarding the self. To fail to adhere to the code is to be a self-deluded, misguided person; to succeed is to be both real and worthy, two spiritual qualities that combine to produce what is called 'authenticity.' (Goffman, 1963: 134–5)

From this followed a partisan attitude of the sociological researcher *vis-à-vis* his or her subject area. In his 1967 Presidential Address to the Society for the Study of Social Problems, Becker urged sociologists to take the side of the deviant. He pictured him as a powerless 'underdog' confronted with an all-powerful society. That people were made into deviants through the very institutions which were to effect their return to normality, meant that society was not democratic. In effect, Becker warned, self-righteousness of the upper-class establishment prevailed whose definitional and disciplinarian powers were used unabashedly. Such stigmatization allowed for individuals to be driven into deviancy by the very mechanisms of its social control. Becker's message was that if veritable humanitarianism was to pervade sociology, it had to give up identifying with society's ruling classes or institutional patterns and embrace identities of the stigmatized ('underdog') instead.

Along these lines of anti-establishment thinking, Eliot Freidson's criticism of professional dominance was a milestone in the medical-sociology literature. In *Profession of Medicine* (1970), he argued that the power of the medical profession consisted of its definitional realm to determine whether or not a symptom was, in fact, pathological or not. He wrote:

> In the sense that medicine had the authority to label one person's complaint an illness and another's complaint not, medicine may be engaged in the *creation of illness as a social state which a human being may assume.* To create illness in this fashion – which may be called socially iatrogenic – is generic to medicine ... Medicine's monopoly includes the right to create illness as an official social role. (Freidson, 1970: 205–6)

In the doctor–patient encounter, Freidson maintained, two equally valid although unequally valued constructions of illness were enacted. On the one side, the dominant medical construction led to treatment which mostly justified itself through the social-control impetus of the physician who labelled a behaviour as illness. Freidson left no doubt that such construction was, to a large extent, self-servingly arbitrary. He wrote:

> Medicine ... is oriented to seeking out and finding illness, which is to say that it seeks to create social meanings of illness where that meaning or that interpretation was lacking before. And insofar as illness is defined as something bad – to be eradicated or contained – medicine plays the role of what Becker called the 'moral entrepreneur.' Medical activity leads to the creation of new rules defining deviance; medical practice seeks to enforce those rules by attracting and treating the newly defined deviant sick. (*ibid.*: 252)

On the other side stood the patient's lay construction of an illness. It was just as credible and convincing as that of a physician, but it was mostly confined to the patient's communications within lay referral networks, that is, influencing or pervading the judgements made in his or her family or work environment. Professional medical work took little notice of patients' construction of their illnesses. Rather, due to its monopoly regarding the realm of health, medicine had power irreconcilable with the public interest, namely, 'the autonomy to define both need and problem and to control their management' (*ibid.*: 331).

British Medical Sociology and the Pathology Framework in the 1970s

In American sociology in the 1960s, the pathology framework was absorbed not only into medical sociology but into the main perspective taken by general sociology. The new name given to the analysis of social pathology was that of labelling theory. Under this title, the substantive fields that had made up the field of social pathology during the first half of the century were re-analysed (e.g. crime, homosexuality, drug addiction, etc.; cf. Weinberg and Rubington, 1968). Goffman's *Asylums* (1961) and *Stigma* (1963), Becker's *Outsiders* (1963) and *The Other Side: Perspectives on Deviance* (1964), and also Scheff's *Being Mentally Ill* (1966), were now icons of a new paradigm pervading general sociology and also became basic texts for medical sociology embracing the idea of labelling and illness careers (see also Gerhardt, 1989, part II).

The introduction of the pathology perspective into medical sociology in Britain dates back to the early 1970s. The conceptual approach was geared toward understanding through empirical data how the labelling processes happened that presumably led to irrevocable careers of illness.

Reality as experienced by the patient in terms of the stages of help-seeking was analysed by David Robinson's *The Process of Becoming Ill* (1971). He found a pre-consultation stage of anticipation and rehearsal of what would be said and done in the consultation, and a post-consultation stage which, indeed, was crucial for whether or not a patient followed a doctor's prescription or advice. A similar structure of patients' reality was shown by Gerry Stimson and Barbara Webb's *Going to See the Doctor* (1975). Interpreting qualitative research material on how women patients experienced their help-seeking, these authors distinguished between five stages of help-seeking. Among them, only the third stage involved doctor–patient contact whereas the later phases consisted of the patient's short-term accounts given to others in the immediate social environment about what had happened in the consultation, and a long-term resolution stage where the outcome of the help-seeking could be compliance with physicians' advice or prescription, but could also be deliberate non-compliance accounted for by a critical opinion about what the consultation had entailed.

Further evidence that patients' reality was at the same time independent of doctors' medical view of illness and consisted of rational sophisticated strategies of coping with intricate life-problems was given by Alan Davis and Gordon Horobin's *Medical Encounters* (1977). It assembled accounts of medical treatment from the perspective of sensitive, bewildered, often powerless patients; they were written by medical sociologists who reported on their own illness experiences. For instance, Nicky Hart described two episodes of puerperal fever and how her physicians refused to believe her correct judgement; Ray Jobling described the intricate rituals of skin care which he, a sufferer from chronic psoriasis, had to go through while a child, and as an adult; and Ann Holohan remembered how she had been treated and what she had felt when she sought medical care because of a complaint which her physician had taken to indicate suspected cancer. These self-reported illness episodes from a patient's point of view were to document how deep a patient's feelings and how rational his or her judgements were as compared with physicians' narrow-minded views of docile and irrational patients. In particular, the book meant to criticize doctors' practice of disregarding or cutting short patients' presentations that often were narratives; because, as was documented through sociologists' accounts, patients' notion of their illnesses represented rich and sensible material denoting their life-worlds and action perspectives. After all, it was with the latter that treatment had to be compatible and it was patients' lives that were affected by, and had to be adapted to, illnesses treated by physicians.

In a similarly medicine-critical vein, Patrick Byrne and Barrie Long's (1976) verbatim documentation of doctor–patient interviews yielded evidence of how little physicians listened to their patients. Other authors found that some negotiation between the physician and the patient regarding the diagnosis as well as the regimen did take place in the medical encounter. But eventually, it was argued, the outcome of the encounter was what had been foreseeable from the medical perspective, dictating a 'hidden agenda' of the doctor–patient interaction. For instance, Philip Strong used tape-recorded interview material from a children's hospital to document that the medical definition of the situation was behind the *Ceremonial Order of the Clinic* (1979). Patrick West, analysing how childhood epilepsy was dealt with in medical consultations, showed how for a varying length of time physicians could refrain from naming the stigmatizing illness or would hesitate to convey the nature of the diagnosis to the parents of a child who had seizures. West wrote:

> Usually the 'diagnosis' constitutes a summary of previously negotiated terms and is in effect a 'quasi-diagnosis' because it is always conditional on the results of the electroencephalogram (EEG) and of the skull X-ray, which are routine procedures used to supplement diagnostic decisions. It is a provisional definition which is potentially open to re-negotiation when additional information has become available. It has parallels with Bloor's analysis of the way 'disposal decisions' about tonsillectomy are delayed until the results of certain investigations are known. (West, 1976: 18)

Michael Bloor (1976a) investigated the variability of criteria used by physicians deciding upon whether or not a child should have adeno-tonsillectomy. He found that far from applying standardized medical knowledge in a diagnosis situation requiring objective judgement, ENT specialists applied widely varying criteria. Therefore, the same condition could in one case be referred to surgery and in another not, depending on which physician made the judgement. In this way, Bloor hinted at the relativity of seemingly objective clinical knowledge. At the same time, he documented how doctors whose decisions often appeared arbitrary nevertheless excluded their patients from influencing the clinical decision. Using tape-recorded data from hospital outpatient encounters, he showed that doctors used three types of routine in order to deny their patients' wishes legitimacy; they were inhibitory, reactive, and reconciliatory routines. About the functions of routines in ENT clinics where most patients were brought by their parents, namely, denial of potential influence, he had this to say:

> Routines can be seen not as simply excluding parents by structuring consultations according to specialists' purposes, but as actively denying parents any potential influence. This process of active denial has been characterised by Lemert (1962) as 'the dynamics of exclusion.' (Bloor, 1976b: 54–5)

Relativity of medical knowledge was the major theme of Robert Dingwall's *Aspects of Illness* (Dingwall, 1976a). He distinguished between illness as a biological reality, and illness as a cultural phenomenon. Whereas the former might indeed be more or less objective malfunctioning, the latter depended on the normative perceptions in a culture or society. Dingwall used cultural anthropology's finding that when an illness affected most people in a primitive population, those who were healthy were excluded due to their apparent deviance. Since illness had a social side that was largely independent of biological pathology, Dingwall maintained, its diagnosis and treatment were not of the objective nature proclaimed by medicine. Rather, medicine consisted of techniques and routines to accomplish the culturally relative definition of a symptom such that it denoted a certain disease; this was done through social routines that were governed by normative rules. In this, he insisted, medicine was not alone. Other professions and semi-professions such as health visiting accomplished their expertise in equally socially constructed ways. He proposed to 'examine the use of the term "profession" by health visitors in relation to their own or other people's behaviour in elaborating "professional" and "non-professional" conduct' (Dingwall, 1976b: 95). Health visitors, he found, consider themselves equal to other professions such as doctors, nurses or social workers; this could be learned from the way in which they talked about themselves *vis-à-vis* the others, and also in that they observed, among other things, 'body management ... as a discriminator between health visiting and other occupations and as an area for conflict over definition of correct performance' (*ibid.*: 100).

These various observations were based, to a large extent, on empirical research conducted under a 'naturalistic' perspective. That is, verbatim transcripts of encounters between professionals and their clients, or data from participant observation in medical settings or from self-descriptions of patients or of health visitors, etc., were used to document what the cognitive perspective was under which those concerned ordered their experienced realities. The aim was to show how in medical encounters those who were not physicians made sense of what went on. Their world-views were claimed to be equally important as those of doctors. The data were interpreted under the assumption that doctors tended to disregard or deny any reality definition different from or competing with their own.

This knowledge interest was common to both volumes of papers originally presented at the 1976 Annual Conference of the British Sociological Association held under the theme of 'Sociology, Health and Illness.' The collection named *Health Care and Health Knowledge* epitomized the view that medical thinking followed relative categories, and that patients' and doctors' views were equally sensible; and the collection entitled *Health and the Division of Labour* held a view of medicine, as Freidson phrased it in the conference's plenary speech, of 'profession as an ideology, as a claim of dedication advanced to protect an interest' (Reid, *et.al.* (eds), 1977: 34). Whereas ideologies also prevailed, for instance, for social workers and clinical psychologists, Nigel Goldie maintained, their influence on professional practice was not the same as that of psychiatrists. That the two non-medical specialities often felt overridden by their medical colleagues in mental hospitals made Goldie question whether a negotiated order prevailed between them. Was not their relationship one of 'imposed order?' One of his non-physician respondents stated the unequal power of medical and non-medical professions by saying about the physician in the psychiatric setting: '"In the treatment of psychiatric illness he is the kingpin. His essential role is to diagnose and delegate treatment in the appropriate way" (3206)' (Goldie, 1977: 147).

One step further went the research focusing on treatment as an interactive production of experienced or negotiated reality (Hall, *et al.*, 1976). Therapeutic communities, for instance, were analysed as venue for joint 'production of facts' as in the research of Rawlings (1981). Investigating – as one of two problems – the issue of success rate, Rawlings came to realize that 'there are no empirical facts to settle such matters .... The way in which members discuss ... "success" may be treated as topic by the researcher and not as problem which it is up to him to solve .... Such a strategy would meet the ethnographic intention of what the organisation is like' (Rawlings, 1981:16) – relinquishing the researcher's role to one of reconstruction of members' (hospital therapists' and patients') ideological views about standards of treatment success.

The assumption was that treatment in hospitals, and to a lesser extent by general practitioners, meant construction if not production of illness through ideological viewpoints deriving from a medical canon of pathology categories. In this way, knowledge meant control over illness realities. Paul Atkinson (1977), explicating 'The Reproduction of Medical Knowledge' in medical school, relied on Michel Foucault's historical relativism to argue that clinical education meant learning practice by 'clinical gaze' (Atkinson, 1977: 83). Atkinson demonstrated 'the orderly and methodic production of clinical facts, and hence of "illness"' (Atkinson, 1981: 103), suggesting:

> Personal experience is used to warrant a stock of knowledge and action in which the clinician places his trust. It can act as the touchstone by which novel events and theories are evaluated .... Illness is constructed in terms of the exclusive expertise of the medical profession. (*ibid.*)

From the vantage point of medicine's identification with clinical ideologies, treatments other than medical interested the sociological observer. Consequently, self-help was proclaimed as an equally viable road to health as medical care. In *Self-Help and Health* (1977), David Robinson and Stuart Henry emphasized that problems such as alcoholism were treated more effectively by self-help than medicine. They took for granted medicine's inadvertent production of illness through treatment ('clinical iatrogenesis'), and they came to criticize even a large number of existing self-help groups in the 1970s for their lack of revolutionary fervour. The latter, to be sure, was to open up a perspective on health divorced from a medicine-related world-view. They wrote, themselves endorsing the view that self-help ought to realize its political potential that made it into something other than medicine's individualist treatment ideology:

> Medicine, as practiced by the medical establishment of developed countries, is increasingly being seen as a major threat to health; not only in the technical sense of malpractice, clinical iatrogenesis and inappropriate treatment, but in the wider political sense of diverting attention from the social-structural and environmental conditions that some would say are the cause of ill-health ... So, are self-help groups the vanguard of the health revolutionaries or the rearguard of the medical establishments? ... At heart, most self-help groups ... operate with the same view of health and illness as conventional helpers. Problems, however they arise, are seen to be the responsibility of the individual. Those self-help groups that look beyond the immediate concerns of their members ... push for recognition of their problem, or for more humane, accessible or competent professional treatment for their problem. Only a minority, like PIE, CHE, the women's groups and Gingerbread, seem to emphasize the distinction between self-help and political actions. (Robinson and Henry, 1977: 123–6)

This opened the door to an emerging sociology of health. Remembering that since the early 1950s Talcott Parsons had taken the view that sociologically health was one of the major focuses of systems formation, Margaret Stacey in the late 1970s revived Parsons' concern. She merged it with the interest of the 1970s in interactionist production of health–illness conceptions. In their overview and reformulation, Stacey and Homans (1978) invoked Marxism, British post-Fabianism, and the work of Eliot Freidson and David Mechanic, beside the approaches which they called phenomenological. They wrote about the latter:

> The increased understanding in sociology of the importance of the actor's point of view has been associated with an increased awareness that sociologists are actors in the society which they are studying and that there are, therefore, strict limits to the extent to which sociology may be said to transcend the values and meanings of the society in which it is practiced. This has had the liberating effect that while, formerly, the sociologist as actor was accused of 'personalizing,' of being anecdotal or idiosyncratic if s/he referred to her/his experiences, now, properly analysed, these are seen to be relevant. (Stacey and Homams, 292)

However, the recommendation to get away from a sociology of medicine and embrace a sociology of health and illness instead was not based on criticism of 'the medical model.' Rather, Stacey and Homans warned that to hold sociology against medicine, juxtaposing an avowed humanist standpoint against a presumed technological bias, was an 'oversimplification … indeed … a misconstruction' of the reality of physicians as social actors (*ibid.*: 292). The conceptual basis for sociology as well as medicine, they thought, was that human suffering should and could be avoided to a considerable extent. Its reduction and maybe elimination were the common interest of the medical as well as social sciences. To understand society thus became part of the medical effort. The healing professions, however, comprised not only physicians but a wide range of caregivers including nurses, midwives, and others. Anticipating the feminism espoused in a later book (Stacey, 1990), medicine inasmuch as it was healing appeared predominantly as an area beyond traditional ideologies since it meant work conducive to females.

The Two Sides of the Dilemma of Social Pathology

Lemert addressed the question of how social pathology came about by adopting Herbert Blumer's adaptation of George Herbert Mead's idea that behaviour is symbolically mediated. Blumer, in the late 1930s, addressed as 'symbolic interactionism' Mead's contribution to the philosophy of pragmatism, that from a behaviourist standpoint a reflexive view of the constitution of self could solve the problem how the social order was situationally produced through significant others, and a generalized other representing society. Lemert, in his 1951 book, responded to the criticism by C. Wright Mills (1943) against the lack of social theory apparent in various previous conceptualizations of social pathology, and he incorporated Blumer's view that 'social interactionism' meant 'naturalistic' research leading to unbiased understanding of social phenomena.

Mills (1943) charged that social pathology – with its focus on personal and social disorganization, and its belief in the possibilities of social reform through educative and welfare-programme efforts – lacked a notion of social structure. In particular, he argued, this deficit kept social pathologists from realizing that inequality which produced poverty, ill-health or crime, was based on the class structure of capitalist society. Since injustice derived from institutional structures, the latter were among the main causes of social pathology, he maintained, and to advocate social change by ameliorative efforts such as education or social work meant to inadvertently condone society's structural ills.

Lemert responded to the criticism by writing a *Social Pathology* that explained how it was through societal reaction that deviance came about. To be sure, he did not adopt the more far-reaching tenets of Mill's political radicalism. But he meant to at least establish a baseline for social theory, accounting for the fact that social pathology came about through deprivation not originating in individual deficiencies but imposed upon the person by societal processes.

As Lemert based his new perspective on Blumer's work, the dilemma contained in Lemert's social pathology view – which is a milestone of medical-sociological understanding of deviance – can be found in Blumer's work, too. Criticism waged against Blumer may also hold for the social pathology viewpoint established in the symbolic interactionist spirit. In his recent book on Blumer, Martyn Hammersley outlined two dilemmas which prevail. One relates to the 'naturalistic' research which Blumer proposed and which was adopted by most later protagonists of the 'neo-Chicagoen' approach – as David Matza (1969) addressed the labelling thesis of Becker, Goffman and Scheff of the 1960s. Hammersley (1989) reconstructs how much Chicago sociology in the 1930s and later relied on the 'naturalistic' approach to show how the definition of the situation of social actors structured their everyday-life problems and solutions. As has been explicated by Barney Glaser and Anselm Strauss's 'Grounded Theory' (1967; cf. Schatzman and Strauss, 1973), the methodological credo was that the researcher was to enter observation of his respondents in their social setting without prior knowledge, as presumptive *tabula rasa.* Any prestructured research question or knowledge interest, they felt, could only distract the researcher's faithful reporting about the observed reality.

Interestingly, Hammersley documents, Blumer believed in the 'naturalistic' approach but also held that the traditional idea was correct that a research design must be formulated, an hypothesis stated, and data analysis conducted that allows for the falsification or verification of hypotheses. Whereas Blumer, as Hammersley shows, on the one hand suggested that established safeguards of objectivity be abandoned in social research he, at the same time, held that these same standards were imperative for scientific evidence. This dilemma, Hammersley maintains, Blumer was never able to solve satisfactorily (Hammersley, 1989: 93).

A similar methodological dilemma prevails in Lemert's work. In *Social Pathology,* he advocated research that documented the 'natural history' of blindness, mental illness, or other forms of deviance.

These were shown to derive from classifications by significant others of a person who subsequently incorporated these labels into the views of his- or herself. In his own research, Lemert (1962) applied the approach to paranoia; he documented through anecdotal material from tape-recorded interviews how people who eventually were diagnosed paranoids were exposed to others' exclusionary practices far exceeding what usually would be expected among colleagues, etc. At the same time, Lemert opted for the life-history as a well-established méthodological approach (Lemert, 1951: 445f.). To be sure, the life-history method had been mainstream in the 1930s and early 1940s (Dollard, 1935; Gottschalck *et al.*, 1945), until after the Second World War the survey became the dominant methodological device of data collection combined with statistical data analysis. It may be noted, however, that Lemert's 'naturalism' – like Blumer's – did not renounce those criteria of objectivity that were to distinguish everyday observations from scientific research. Although naïvety, so to speak, guided the 'naturalistic' strategy, the credo was that the outcome of observation and data analysis ought to be systematic knowledge which could only derive from intersubjectively valid research.

The latter's guarantors differed for later authors adopting qualitative methodology; but most of them accepted the necessity of some kind of criteria for the objectivity of the interpretation. For instance, in *Theoretical Sensitivity*, Glaser (1978) claimed that 'grounded-theory methodology' achieved intersubjective validity of data interpretation by creating impressions of plausibility in the reader of a research report. In the same vein, William J. Filstead's compendium summarizing the 'new' methodology of the 1960s, *Qualitative Methodology: Firsthand Involvement With the Social World*, devoted a part to the 'Problems of Validity and Reliability,' and Robert Emerson's *Field Research* (1983) did likewise.

The other dilemma of Blumer, Hammersley shows, is that whereas he based his work on the writings of George Herbert Mead, he inadvertently discarded or abandoned most of Mead's theoretical assumptions.

Hammersley cites the view of C. McPhail and C. Rexroat (1979) that Blumer's work suffers from an 'ontological paradox,' namely,

> a conflict between his realist account of the process of research in which the nature of the world is discovered, and, using my terms, the phenomenalism of symbolic interactionism, in which meanings are portrayed as constructions, not reflections of some independent reality. (Hammersley, 1989: 194)

The issue, then, is the ontological status of constructions. When Peter Berger and Thomas Luckmann analysed *The Social Construction of Reality* (1966), they assumed that behaviour necessarily was steeped in routinized stocks of knowledge representing internalized and externalized institutional rules. Whereas they identified these rules with agents who stood for institutionalized collective definitions of reality, Freidson in *Profession of Medicine* added an element of uncontrolled power to the role of such agents. For him, construction of illness reality by medicine meant power-prone moral entrepreneurship to carve out a realm of unchecked domination. He wrote:

> I have been stimulated by Berger and Luckmann, who declare that 'reality is socially defined. But the definitions are always *embodied,* that is, concrete individuals and groups of individuals serve as definers of reality. To understand the state of the socially constructed universe at any given time, or its change over time, one must understand the social organization that permits the definers to do their defining.' The consulting profession's position of organized autonomy, which includes its monopoly over special work, and its special place in the social order, permits the profession to create an important segment of the socially constructed universe. What it creates is composed of its relatively reliable knowledge, its sense of mission, and its practical institutions. The substance of those creations arises from the experience of the creators. The experience of the creators is a function of the perspective they have gained by virtue of being in an especially protected, autonomous position in the social structure, a position which systematically discounts the experience and evaluation of the laymen outside. (Freidson, 1970: 379–80)

It is from this vantage point that Freidson deplored 'social iatrogenics,' that is, the creation of illness labels by medicine proceeding to treat patients for illnesses whose definition it controls monopolistically. The sociologist, accordingly, was to reveal the *relativity* of social construction by exposing self-serving interests behind apparently altruistic practices.

The relativity issue has been discussed by various authors. In the early 1940s, Fuller introduced relativity between the normal and the abnormal; he wanted to replace the overtone of righteousness in the earlier social pathology literature with a scientific standpoint allowing for, in Max Weber's terms, value neutrality. Lemert, in his *Social Pathology* (1951), distinguished between deviance and the deviant, using the relativity idea to prove that deviance developed through a social process which, in principle, could happen to anyone – which meant that the label represented injustice epitomized by deprivation and exclusion. Goffman introduced the notion of contingency to account for the diagnosis of mental illness or other deviances of the person; he found that wilful or inadvertent discrimination accompanied the treatment that therefore produced rather than cured the person's state of deviation. Bloor, in the 1970s, for instance, discovering that no fixed relationship existed between symptoms and diagnosis, concluded that medical knowledge was relative and the medical profession might better be deprived of its unquestioned authority. In a similar vein, Robinson and Henry's plea for self-help instead of medical treatment implied that the former was equivalent, if not preferable, to the latter.

The relativity stance as part of the analysis of social construction claims scientific dignity. Its opposition to medicine's presumed political interests that are contained in medical knowledge, invokes humanism in sociology. When Becker (1967) divided the world into an array of value-laden standpoints, he demanded the sociologist's identification with the standpoint of the weak. Such self-styled humanism has pervaded the discussion of social construction in medical sociology.

Its dilemma lies in theoretical assumptions making for an 'ontological paradox.' As humanist discipline, social pathology-prone medical sociology proclaims the relativity of illness labels. It denies justification to stigma or deprivation that could follow from or is brought about by a diagnostic or therapeutic measure. The person, in this vein, is an holistic human being whose authenticity is, in principle, unaffected by anything done to him or her by societal agencies.

Accordingly, medicine is a societal agency doing diagnosis or treatment to the individual who, from this standpoint, would be better off if he or she were left alone. Anything done by societal agencies, in this vein, can only curtail the rights and freedoms of the authentic person. The theoretical view of society invoked by this approach is that of 'vexacious fact.' In his criticism of sociology's presumably hermetic image of oversocialized man, Ralf Dahrendorf, using the metaphor that society is a 'vexacious fact,' contrasted it with the person whose freedom should be preserved or at least postulated by the sociologist. When analysing *homo sociologicus* (1958/1973), Dahrendorf maintained, sociologists should be aware of the dichotomy between social constraints representing the hermetic reality of society as 'vexacious fact,' and individual freedom. This suggested a dichotomy between power that was lodged with society and freedom that was lodged with the individual.

This dichotomous image of the society–individual relationship is invoked by the thesis that deviance is but social construction making for stigmatization of the 'underdog.' Research based on this idea of society–individual antagonism may misjudge reality when presumably it *discovers* all-pervasive social construction that prevails in medical and other work. The dilemma in which social pathology-related medical sociology finds itself is that, at the same time, the society individual dichotomy is endorsed and the claim is made that empirical reality of medical life-worlds can be observed in an objective way, yielding data about the nature of the practice of medicine.

Beneath and Beyond the Dilemma

When, in the early 1940s, the analysis of social pathology established its scientific status by addressing the relativity of deviance, a second line of thought was introduced that was not followed up after the Second World War. Fuller's idea that the same social processes explained the normal and the deviant was taken up by Brown's *Social Pathology* (1942) and became common knowledge through Lemert's *Social Pathology* (1951), but the more contemporaneous applications discussed by Brown were not preserved in what ten years later became labelling theory.

Brown hinted at German fascism when he discussed 'social epidemics.' He thereby implied that societies existed to which the label of social pathology could be applied more easily than to others whose structure was more democratic. He castigated the Führer principle of social domination, emphasizing that National Socialism was based on pathological mechanisms far more pervasive than in the contemporary USA.

This distinction was not preserved in Lemert's conception of symbolic processes making for sociopathic behaviour and identities. The topic of political pathology was discussed by Brown and also some of the earlier approaches to social pathology, e.g. when Gillin addressed 'pathology of the state' epitomizing legislation that discriminated against parts of the population, etc. But Lemert abandoned this comprehensive perspective on social pathology and instead concentrated on the social processes of becoming a deviant. Only in his incorporating political radicalism into the realm of topics of social pathology did the discussion of the political sphere by earlier approaches find a relatively weak follow-up. Besides, since

Lemert's knowledge interest is to reveal the relativity of social construction of labels, political radicalism appears as just another label and is not judged according to the realistic dangers it harbours for democratic state and society.

It was from this relativistic angle that Goffman, Becker and Scheff resumed the discussion in the 1960s. They realized that if sociology failed to distinguish between democratic (normal) and fascist (pathological) society, anti-humanism could ensue. On this basis, they reintroduced the option for non-pathological society by endorsing the sick or deviant individual's unaffected humaneness. They claimed that deprivation and stigma of the 'underdog' was the social pathology which sociology ought to combat.

British medical sociology, partly inspired by Freidson's plea that patients' constructions of illness were as viable as those of doctors, followed in the footsteps of labelling theory's idea of the political. Whereas empirical societies in the 1960s were not analysed as more or less pathological – as could have been done, for instance, judging pathological the totalitarian state and society in the Soviet Union – society *as such* was understood to be pathological and to produce pathologies. It was argued that constructions of pathology served the interests of the ruling establishment, medical or otherwise. In other words, whereas social pathology was analysed as an outcome of ubiquitous processes of power and privilege and was found preferably in Western societies, Eastern non-democratic societies were rarely included in the analysis and their systems of repression were not identified with social pathology.

The failure of the social pathology literature, including that of medical sociology, to distinguish between pathological and non-pathological social systems might have been avoided. In 1942, writing about *Propaganda and Social Control*, Talcott Parsons found two types of social control. One was integration of society through voluntary conformity of members with community norms accepted through insight and commitment. The principle of such democratic social structure was reciprocity in the relationships between individuals. Deviance, if it occurred, was remedied by medical practice insulating the person from others and guiding him or her back to recovery through disinterested professional therapy. The other type of social control was repressive. It produced society's functioning by forcing the individuals to comply with rules that themselves could call for, rather than discourage, deviance. The latter, to be sure, meant mental illness, such as paranoia or neuroses, and criminality. In somewhat abstract terms, Parsons distinguished between a society that curtailed mental aberrations in the 'definition of the situation' – such as racist anti-Semitism – and a society that exacerbated such deviance. He wrote:

> Every social system, functionally regarded, faces a control problem on the level of overt behavior … The direct obverse of the functional necessity of integration is the existence of many important tendencies and seeds of deviant behavior … It seems to be inherent in the structure of human action that there are, fundamentally, two kinds of channels through which 'pressure' to control behavior may be exerted … On the one hand, the appeal may be to what psychoanalysts call the 'reality principle,' and the mechanism will then operate through the actual or potential alteration of the situation in which people act … On the other hand, appeal will be made to the 'state of mind' or the 'sentiments' of the actor relatively independently of potential alterations in the situation in which he acts … It is in this latter category that propaganda falls, as one important mechanism for controlling action – not of course necessarily in the interest of checking deviant tendencies, quite possibly of promoting them. (Parsons, 1942/1954: 148–9)

The latter, to be sure, meant pathological or, as Parsons called it, *deviant society*. In his *Social System* (1951), he further elaborated on the distinction between integrated (democratic) and deviant (fascist) society. However, the idea was rarely recognized behind his abstract terminology. To be sure, Chapter X uses medical practice – described as the ideal type that defines democratic, non-pathological society – in order to give an example of how pathology is effectively and humanely checked by the medical profession embracing disinterested service to the suffering patient.

Beyond the dilemma of social pathology, I wish to argue, is the idea that societies may be pathological, or may be democratic. Not that the latter are idealized or should be without fault or, in fact, would lack pathological tendencies such as disregard for humaneness or humanity. But to distinguish between fascist and democratic societies saves medical sociology, and indeed sociology, from making unrealistic claims regarding society's balance between freedom and necessity. This may help to avoid denouncing existing democracies on the grounds that they fall short of overambitious ideals. To be on the side of the 'underdog,' then, means to distinguish between realistic and unrealistic construction of medical and other labels. It also means that it is not politically suspect to acknowledge that illness, in fact, exists as a reality and must be treated competently by physicians.

References

- Atkinson, Paul, 'The Reproduction of Medical Knowledge,' in Robert Dingwall, Christian Heath, Margaret Reid and Margaret Stacey (eds), *Health Care and Health Knowledge* (London: Croom Helm, 1977), 85–106.
- Atkinson, Paul, *The Clinical Experience. The Construction and Reconstruction of Medical Reality* (London: Gower, 1981).
- Becker, Howard, *Outsiders: Studies in the Sociology of Deviance* (New York: Free Press, 1963).
- Becker, Howard, *The Other Side: Perspectives on Deviance* (New York: Collier Macmillan, 1964).
- Becker, Howard, 'Whose Side Are We On?,' *Social Problems*, 14 (1967), 239–47.
- Berger, Peter L. and Luckmann, Thomas, *The Social Construction of Reality. A Treatise in the Sociology of Knowledge* (New York: Doubleday, 1966).
- Bloor, Michael, 'Professional Autonomy and Client Exclusion: A Study of ENT Clinics,' in Michael Wadsworth and David Robinson (eds), *Studies in Everyday Medical Life* (London: Martin Robertson, 1976a), 52–68.
- Bloor, Michael, 'Bishop Berkeley and the Adenotonsillectomy Enigma: An Exploration of Variation in the Social Construction of Medical Disposals,' *Sociology*, 10 (1976b), 43–61.
- Blumer, Herbert, *Symbolic Interactionism* (Berkeley: University of California Press, 1969).
- Brown, Lawrence Guy, *Social Pathology. Personal and Social Disorganization* (New York: F. S. Crofts Co., 1942).
- Byrne, Patrick S. and Long, Barrie E. L., *Doctors Talking To Patients. A Study of Verbal Behaviour of General Practitioners Consulting in Their Surgeries* (London: HMSO, 1976).
- Dahrendorf, Ralf, *Homo Sociologicus* (London: Routledge & Kegan Paul, 1973; originally in German, 1958).
- Davis, Alan and Horobin, Gordon (eds), *Medical Encounters* (London: Croom Helm, 1977).
- Dingwall, Robert, *Aspects of Illness* (London: Martin Robertson, 1976a).
- Dingwall, Robert, (in Wadsworth and Robinson 1976b)
- Dingwall, Robert, Heath, Christian, Reid, Margaret and Stacey, Margaret (eds), *Health Care and Health Knowledge* (London: Croom Helm, 1977).
- Dollard, John, *Criteria for the Life History* (New Haven: Yale University Press, 1935).

- Emerson, Robert (ed.), *Field Research* (Boston: Little, Brown, 1983).
- Filstead, William J. (ed.), *Qualitative Methodology* (Chicago: Markham, 1970).
- Freidson, Eliot, *Profession of Medicine. A Study of the Sociology of Applied Knowledge* (New York: Dodd, Mead, 1970).
- Freidson, Eliot, 'The Futures of Professionalization,' in Margaret Stacey, Margaret Reid, Christian Heath and Robert Dingwall (eds), *Health and the Division of Labour* (London: Croom Helm, 1977), 14–40.
- Fuller, Richard C., *Social Pathology* (New York: 1940a).
- Fuller, Richard C. and Myers, Richard R., 'Some Aspects of a Theory of Social Problems,' *American Sociological Review*, 6 (1941), 24–32.
- Gerhardt, Uta, *Ideas About Illness. An Intellectual and Political History of Medical Sociology* (London: Macmillan, 1989).
- Gerhardt, Uta (ed.), *Talcott Parsons on National Socialism* (New York: Aldine de Gruyter, 1993).
- Gillin, John L., *Social Pathology* (New York: The Century, 1933; revised 2nd edition 1939; revised 3rd edition 1946: New York: Appleton Century).
- Gillin, John L. and Blackmar, Frank W., *Outlines of Sociology* (New York: Macmillan, 1930).
- Glaser, Barney, *Theoretical Sensitivity* (Mill Valley: Sociology Press, 1978).
- Glaser, Barney and Strauss, Anselm, *The Discovery of Grounded Theory* (Chicago: Aldine de Gruyter, 1967).
- Goffman, Erving, *Asylums: Essays on the Social Situation of Mental Patients and Other Inmates* (New York: Doubleday, 1961).
- Goffman, Erving, *Stigma: Notes on the Management of Spoiled Identity* (Englewood Cliffs, N.J.: Prentice Hall, 1963).
- Goldie, Nigel, 'The Division of Labour Among the Health Professions – A Negotiated or an Imposed Order?,' in Margaret Stacey, Margaret Reid, Christian Heath and Robert Dingwall (eds), *Health and the Division of Labour* (London: Croom Helm, 1977), 141–64.
- Gottschalck, Louis, Kluckhohn, Clyde and Angell, Robert, *The Use of Personal Documents in History, Anthropology, and Sociology* (New York: Social Science Research Council, 1945).
- Hall, David, Pill, Roisin and Clough, Fred, 'Notes for a Conceptual Model of Hospital Experiences as an Interactive Process,' in Margaret Stacey (ed.), *The Sociology of the NHS* (Keele: Sociological Review Monographs No. 22, 1976), 142–55.
- Hammersley, Martyn, *The Dilemma of Qualitative Method* (London: Routledge, 1989).

- Lemert, Edwin, *Social Pathology* (New York: McGraw-Hill, 1951).
- Lemert, Edwin, 'Paranoia and the Dynamics of Exclusion,' *Sociometry*, 25 (1962), 2–20.
- Mangold, George B., *Social Pathology* (New York: Macmillan, 1932; 2nd edition 1934).
- Matza, David, *Becoming Deviant* (Englewood Cliffs, N. J.: Prentice Hall, 1969).
- McPhail, C. and Rexroat, C., 'Mead vs. Blumer: The Divergent Methodological Perpectives of Social Behaviorism and Symbolic Interactionism,' *American Sociological Review*, 44 (1979), 449–67.
- Mills, C. Wright, 'The Professional Ideology of Social Pathologists,' *American Journal of Sociology*, 49 (1943), 165–80.
- Parsons, Talcott, 'Propaganda and Social Control,' *Psychiatry*, 5 (1942), 551–72 (reprinted in *Essays in Sociological Theory*, rev. edn New York: Macmillan, 1954, 142–76).
- Parsons, Talcott, *The Social System* (Glencoe, Ill.: The Free Press, 1951).
- Queen, Stuart A. and Mann, Delbert M., *Social Pathology* (New York: Thomas Y. Crowell, 1925; 2nd edition 1936).
- Queen, Stuart A. and Gruener, Jennette R., *Social Pathology: Obstacles to Social Participation* (New York: Thomas Y. Crowell, 1940).
- Rawlings, Barbara, 'The Production of Facts in a Therapeutic Community,'in Paul Atkinson and Christian Heath (eds), *Medical Work. Realities and Routines* (London: Gower, 1981), 1–18.
- Robinson, David, *The Process of Becoming Ill* (London: Routledge & Kegan Paul, 1971).
- Robinson, David and Henry, Stuart, *Self-Help and Health. Mutual Aid for Mutual Problems* (London: Martin Robertson, 1977).
- Schatzman, Leonard and Strauss, Anselm L., *Field Research: Strategies of Natural Research* (Englewood Cliffs, N. J.: Prentice Hall, 1973).
- Scheff, Thomas, *Being Mentally Ill: A Sociological Theory* (Chicago: Aldine de Gruyter, 1966).
- Stacey, Margaret, *Women and Healing* (1990).
- Stacey, Margaret and Homans, Hilary, 'The Sociology of Health and Illness: Its Present State, Future Prospects and Potential for Health Research,' *Sociology*, 12 (1978), 281–307.
- Stacey, Margaret, Reid, Margaret, Heath, Christian and Dingwall, Robert (eds), *Health and the Division of Labour* (London: Croom Helm, 1977).
- Stimson, Gerry and Webb, Barbara, *Going to See the Doctor* (London: Routledge & Kegan Paul, 1975).
- Strecker, Edward, *Beyond the Clinical Frontiers. A Psychiatrist Views*

Crowd Behavior (New York: Norton, 1940).

- Strong, Philip M., *The Ceremonial Order of the Clinic. Parents, Doctors, and Medical Bureaucracies* (London: Routledge & Kegan Paul, 1979).
- Weinberg, Earl and Rubington, Martin (eds), *Deviance: The Interactionist Perspective* (New York: Macmillan, 1968).
- West, Patrick, 'The Physician and the Management of Childhood Epilepsy,' in Michael Wadsworth and David Robinson (eds), *Studies in Everyday Medical Life* (London: Martin Robertson, 1976), 13–31.

7

The Social Space of Illness

David Armstrong

Introduction

How does a new medical speciality emerge? According to Adam Smith in *The Wealth of Nations* (1776) it is the economic imperative which produces a division of labour to maximize productivity. Thus, medical practitioners have often searched out a protected economic niche by taking a special interest in a particular part of the human body: Peterson has suggested that this economic motive was important in nineteenth-century specialization in England (Peterson, 1978) and Stevens, similarly, in twentieth-century America (Stevens, 1971).

However, the economic model only offers a partial explanation of the medical division of labour. In part, this is because the subdivision of a task that characterizes the classical division of labour is largely absent from medicine. Doctors rarely specialize in diagnosis or treatment alone; rather, as Rosen observed, the medical practitioner tends to create a total rather than a partial product (Rosen, 1944). What differentiates speciality from speciality is the accentuation placed on a component of the task: it is this emphasis, he suggests, rather than a complete separation which distinguishes medical specialization from the broader health division of labour.

The medical profession's own explanation of speciality formation has also tended to eschew economic factors and stress the importance of the 'natural growth' of knowledge. Medical knowledge was believed to be organic, growing and differentiating apparently of its own accord. Thus the cognitive base of medicine was seen as constantly expanding and then, amoeba-like, fragmenting. 'The evolution of medicine,' noted Russell Brain in 1953, 'has involved a process of differentiation, which has some parallel with, and been intimately related to the increase in knowledge' (Brain, 1953: 959) or as Henry

Cohen observed, 'advancing knowledge must inevitably lead to specialisation in all fields' (Cohen, 1960: 9). Such a cognitive model also underpins Stevens' classic account of medical specialization in Britain: 'the search for new knowledge,' she claimed, 'the pursuit of greater efficiency and excellence, and an increasing public faith in expertise in all walks of life encouraged doctors to develop exclusive interests and to set themselves up as specialists in their chosen field ... Specialisation was prompted by those who sought excellence in particular areas within an expanding field; it was an inevitable and desirable accompaniment of scientific advance.' (Stevens, 1966: 3)

Yet whatever its basis – and whatever its contemporary explanation – the emergence of new disciplines in medicine has occurred within a well-defined framework. As Rosen observed, it was only in Ancient Egypt and during the last two centuries that specialization has existed to an appreciable degree, a phenomenon he linked specifically to contemporary theories of the body (Rosen, 1944). In short, specialization has only occurred historically when the prevailing system of medicine has compartmentalized the body. Thus, with the change at the turn of the eighteenth century from the notion of disease as a humoral systemic disorder to a localized pathological lesion (Foucault, 1973), medical practitioners could concentrate on one locality and thus become specialists of diseases of the heart, eye, chest, etc. The modern belief that the body is divisible, or at least analysable, into parts would therefore seem an important conceptual precondition for medical specialization. In other words, the separate existence of, say, cardiology and neurology presupposes an analytic distinction – perhaps in structure and/or function – between cardiovascular and neurological systems in the body (Armstrong, 1993a).

In summary, the conceptual model of illness underpinning the system of clinical practice that first emerged at the end of the eighteenth century involved the identification of the pathological lesion through the inferential techniques of the clinical examination. These techniques were deployed to analyse the three-dimensional volume of the body wherein the disease was hidden. In these circumstances specialization was related largely to subdivisions of the space or 'volume' of the body. However, this account of the emergence of new specialities in medicine does not provide a framework for understanding the development of social medicine; on the contrary, this account provides a description of a primary differentiation process to which, importantly, social medicine did not belong. Social medicine was different precisely because it was not directly related to the analysis of corporal space.

Social Medicine

Social medicine might claim some parentage in the nineteenth-century public health movement. However, despite the apparent environmental concerns of the latter, it too, like the contemporary branches of clinical medicine, was firmly focused on the three-dimensional volume of the human body. The task of nineteenth-century public health was to sanitize the boundary which separated body from non-body (or nature). All matter which crossed this boundary, whether inward as food, water and air, or outward as bodily wastes, were subjected to rigorous monitoring. The effect of these practices was to delineate even more clearly the margin and limits of the three-dimensional volume of the body in which clinical medicine searched for its elusive lesion. From food inspection to miasmatic dangers, from oral hygiene to preoccupation with constipation, from effluent disposal to removal of the dead, nineteenth-century public health deployed a web of surveillance around the well-defined contours of the living body (Armstrong, 1993b).

Early in the twentieth century a new perspective on the nature of illness began to emerge. This new vision continued nineteenth-century public health's techniques of hygiene but they were directed at a new object – not the dangers that lurked around body boundaries, but the threats that haunted a space defined by the relationships between bodies. This new interpersonal hygiene, as it was called, identified other people as the health hazard, not the ubiquitous dirt of the previous century. For example, in the early years of the twentieth century tuberculosis was reclassified into a disease of contagion rather than poor sanitary conditions; venereal disease, though it might exist in the body of an individual patient, was perceived as constantly moving between sexual contacts; and the school medical service began its never-ending task to exclude contagion and promote interpersonal hygiene amongst schoolchildren: 'The school child, easily seen, easily examined, easily described has enabled us to crystallise the conception of personal hygiene and to test the possibilities of remedial measures.' (Mackenzie, 1906: 510)

At the same time as these reformulations in the nature and form of physical illnesses, the field of psychiatric disease was also reorganized. From an exclusive emphasis in the nineteenth century on the problems of insanity, the new psychological medicine began to address the problems of the neuroses: the neuroses affected everyone and were seen to be linked to relationships, both current and past. As with the new interpersonal hygiene, it was the interstices of the social that harboured the germ of mental problems and these could only be combated by a rigorous mental hygiene (Armstrong, 1983).

The space between bodies that interpersonal hygiene targeted was in part the physical space across which contagious organisms passed; but it was also a space of relationships because, by and large, the anonymous, unknown contact was less frequent and therefore less dangerous than contacts with friends and relatives. Thus, the techniques of interpersonal hygiene had as their object the interpersonal space between bodies. And as the new hygienic techniques were gradually extended, they had the effect of further crystallizing and clarifying the nature of this embryonic conceptual space. It was the consolidation of this space that led to interpersonal hygiene being transposed into social medicine in the inter-war years (Sand, 1952).

In his overview of the emergence of social medicine, Sand located its first appearance firmly to the early years of the twentieth century with the advent of socio-clinical medicine, industrial medicine, insurance medicine, preventive medicine, and social hygiene. Despite a professorial chair in Germany in 1902, the new discipline was only acknowledged in Britain about the time of the Second World War. In this latter period, claimed Sand, the principles of social medicine paid dividends in terms of increased production and improved standards of general health. These principles embraced 'aptitude tests in the recruiting of labour, the fighting forces and auxiliary services, civil as well as military; systematic training for the work proposed; rehabilitation of the disabled; rational distribution of foodstuffs; extra health protection, particularly for workers, expectant mothers and children; organization of leisure activities; and development and improvement of social services.'

The history of the formalization of social medicine in Britain is very much intertwined with the life of John Ryle who, after a distinguished career as an academic general physician, 'changed disciplines' to move to Oxford to be the first professor of social medicine in a newly established Institute of Social Medicine (Ryle, 1948). But the outline of the new social medicine in Britain had begun to appear many years earlier as interpersonal hygiene extended its domain. Even the Royal College of Physicians felt moved to set up a Social and Preventive Medicine Committee in 1942 to prepare for the development of a subject that offered 'a relatively novel point of view.' The Report of the Interdepartmental Committee on Medical

Schools, chaired by Sir William Goodenough and published in 1944, acknowledged that social medicine 'signifies a particular conception of Medicine; a conception that regards the promotion of health as a primary duty of the doctor, that pays heed to man's social environment and heredity as they affect health, and that recognizes that personal problems of health and sickness may have communal as well as individual aspects.'

In summary, social medicine was the hygienic regime which sought to manage dangers from the space between bodies. It did not engage with an isolated physical body, nor indeed a simple collection of those same bodies; social medicine recognized the interactions of those bodies as the locus of illness and as the space for intervention. Whereas other medical specialities that emerged during the twentieth century reflected the increasing fragmentation of the body and the search for the internal pathological lesion, the growth of social medicine tracked the unfolding of psychosocial space. The appearance of this new conceptual space early in the twentieth century was also accompanied by the emergence of other, parallel, 'new' disciplines. For example, psychology and sociology brought to bear their own precise methodological techniques for the exploration of this novel universe. And clustered around this new psychosocial space alliances began to emerge: psychology readily formed its compact with medicine, particularly in the forms of the new medical psychology and psychological medicine. This alliance added the psychosocial characteristics of individual difference to the anatomical identity of sanitary science. The links between medicine and sociology were slower to emerge, but after the Second World War a number of health problems were identified by the newly invigorated social medicine which demanded closer collaboration with sociologists.

Medical Sociology

Medical sociology emerged after the Second World War as a realization of further disciplinary consolidation in the relatively novel social space of illness. A strategy of social hygiene brought into focus a number of new problems that sociology might help address. Illness was no longer simply a corporal lesion, but a characteristic of a community, and its identification did not demand the clinical method but the techniques of the survey. Surveys, such as the War-time Social Survey in Britain or the 9,000-family periodic health canvas in the USA (Collins *et al.*, 1933), helped map the extent of illness in the community.

But of particular significance for the growth of medical sociology was the transformation of the patient. Under a system of pathological medicine, the patient was no more than the repository of the lesion; but early in the twentieth century the patient as actor was recognized in regimes of personal hygiene and in concerns for patient 'defaulters' from treatment, particularly from that of venereal disease. By the middle of the century health education was firmly established as an essential part of the public health programme. 'Health authorities,' wrote Derryberry in 1945, 'are becoming increasingly aware that many diseases are uncontrollable without the active participation of the people themselves.' Whereas a few decades earlier the community was only involved in public health insofar as their electoral or political support was required, now people had to be involved from the very beginning of any programme because they themselves were the agents of health practice (Derryberry, 1949).

A further major point for the articulation of ideas on patient behaviour appeared in April 1955 in the USA when the Salk vaccine was declared safe and an effective protection against poliomyelitis. A national vaccination programme commenced at once and became the new focus on the problems of participation within the contemporary public health literature. Here for once was a programme with undeniable benefits yet which the public failed to support wholeheartedly.

What were the public's attitudes towards vaccination? What factors precluded their involvement? Indeed the questions began even before the vaccine was proved to be safe and effective. Clausen and his colleagues noted in their report on parental reactions to the vaccine trials that they 'may be useful in indicating in somewhat greater detail than is usually available the factors influencing participation in such a program and the attitude and characteristics of participants and non-participants .... Using the technics of social science research, it would seem fruitful to investigate further the methods of reaching and influencing those segments of the population which tend to be non-participants in such public health programs.' (Clausen *et al.*, 1954)

In similar fashion, response to community X-ray services for tuberculosis and to the new multi-phasic screening programmes focused attention on patient behaviour (Hochbaum, 1956).

Whereas during the early part of the century human behaviour had seemed to be governed by instinct, that is from a fixed biological point, during the late 1950s public health discovered beliefs as the mainspring of human action. The theories of Rosenstock *et al.* of 1959 of why people failed to seek polio vaccination had become, by 1965, the basis for a more generalized model of health beliefs and focus on patient activity (Rosenstock, 1965).

One of the effects of the recruitment of the patient as an integral component of health management was the change in the status and nature of 'patient' identity. Parsons' notion of the sick-role – one of the earliest programmatic statements for the new discipline of medical sociology – prefigured this concern in its identification of an active patient and a social dimension to illness (Parsons, 1951). In the past the transition from person-status to patient-status had been marked by 'coming under the doctor.' In the new regime patienthood began to lose its old meaning: the boundary between healthy person and patient became problematic. This shift was marked by the extension of patient status (or at least potential status) as everyone came under medical/health surveillance through the gradual recruitment of everyone to the medical enterprise. A number of post-war health surveys confirmed that a rigid distinction between health and illness was meaningless: everyone had health problems, everyone was 'at risk health care merely touched the tip of the morbidity iceberg (Last, 1963).

In 1960 Mechanic and Volkart introduced the concept of 'illness behaviour' to explain the decision-making process whereby a person with symptoms became a patient with illness. Illness behaviour was another component of the post-war fascination with the weakening person–patient interface. The transition from person to patient did not signify the simple and absolute distinction between health and illness; people made their own personal judgements and decisions about illness – a judgement that might well not accord with medical opinion.

A further indication of this transformation of patienthood was marked by the sudden interest in the placebo effect from about 1948 (Shapiro, 1960). The placebo effect could not exist prior to this time because medicine could see only a passive body; recognition of the placebo effect revealed the moment when subjective mental processes began to seize control of the body. In parallel, medicine discovered the doctor–patient relationship as a new and problematic topic (Armstrong, 1982). The relationship was not only between practitioner and body as of old, but also between practitioner and subjective mind: doctors consulted as much with their patients as 'agents' as with their patients as bodies.

New Space, New Disciplines

So what are the implications of this analysis for the relationship between social medicine and medical sociology? Under a system of clinical medicine based on the corporal pathological lesion, specialization is largely predicated on the subdivisions of the human body. If both social medicine and medical sociology crystallized in a novel illness space, what are the commensurate 'fracture points' in the new space of the social? The social itself seems less intuitively divisible than the body. This might suggest that different definitions of the social and the nature of this space are more likely to delineate and separate disciplines colonizing this cognitive domain.

In 1974 the old public health/social medicine was given the new title of community medicine. Community medicine has itself been replaced recently by the new discipline of public health medicine. Besides its specific role in the operation of the purchaser-provider function in the reformed NHS, what is the focus of this new speciality? The concerns of the 'new public health medicine' are less the socio-physical spaces between bodies and more the abstracted products of social activities in the form through which they feed back and jeopardize health status. Thus, for example, damage to the ozone layer, pollutants in the air, contaminants in food and water, radiation from nuclear facilities, etc., prove the essential dangers of the late twentieth century (Armstrong, 1993b). This perspective unifies the environmental concerns of nineteenth-century public health with the social analysis of the twentieth century: a commitment to an ecological politics that encompasses both the natural and the social.

Medical sociology has taken a different route. In its study of social factors in the origins of disease it is the legitimate successor to social medicine: it remains social space, particularly in the form of relationships, which somehow harbour and engender illness. In addition, it has added a novel perspective to this illness of social spaces: in an extension of its concerns with patient behaviour it has begun to pursue the experience of illness by a social subject. Thus, whereas the new public health has sought to integrate social and natural space, medical sociology has attempted a synthesis of social and subjective. However, for both disciplines the social remains the seminal space of illness.

Conclusion

For a traditional form of medical history the answer to the question of what brings about the emergence of new disciplines is bound up with a notion of progress. It is advance in science that leads to the discovery of new areas, and further division of labour in the medical task; it is the technological breakthrough which produces a new device or technique around which a new speciality crystallizes; it is the emergence of a new disease, or set of diseases, that elicits a response in terms of migration to a new discipline. A constant feature of these accounts is that the field of study exists separate from and essentially prior to the emergence of the workers who come to form the discipline.

Thus, insofar as medicine is concerned, diseases existed in nature before the practice of medicine was organized as a discrete professional area of work; it is the struggle to combat disease which elicits an organized response that, in its turn, coalesces into a formal discipline.

The argument of this chapter is that medical specialities can better be seen as clustering around a particular space in which notions of health and illness reside. For most of medicine – and for most medical specialities – this has been the three-dimensional volume of the human body, but during the twentieth century a new space of health/illness has unfolded in which new disciplines have crystallized: social medicine and medical sociology both belong to this epistemological transformation.

References

- Armstrong, D., 'Child Development and Medical Ontology,' *Social Science and Medicine,* 13, (1979), 9–12.
- Armstrong, D., 'The Doctor–Patient Relationship: 1930–1980,' in P. Wright and A. Treacher (eds), *TheProblem of Medical Knowledge* (Edinburgh: Edinburgh University Press, 1982).
- Armstrong, D., *Political Anatomy of the Body: Medical Knowledge in Britain in theTwentieth Century* (Cambridge: Cambridge University Press, 1983).
- Armstrong, D., 'The Medical Division of Labour in E. Messer-Davidow, Shumway, D. R. and Sylvan, D. J. (eds), *Knowledges: Historical and Critical Studies in Disciplinarity* (Charlottesville: University of Virginia Press, 1993a).
- Armstrong, D., 'Public Health Spaces and the Fabrication of Identity,' *Sociology,* 27 (1993b), 393–410.
- Brain, R., 'The Need for a Philosophy of Medicine,' *Lancet,* 1 (1953), 959–64.
- Clausen, J. A. *et al.*, 'Parent Attitudes Towards Participation of Their Children in Polio Vaccine Trials', *American Journal of Public Health,* 44 (1954), 1526.
- Cohen, H., 'Reflections on Specialization in Medicine *Annals of the Royal College of Surgeons,* 27 (1960), 1–13.
- Collins, S. D. *et al.*, 'Causes of Illness in 9000 Families Based on Nationwide Periodic Canvasses, 1928–31,' *Public Health Reports,* 48 (1933), 283.
- Derryberry, M., 'Health Education in the Public Health Program,' *Public Health Reports,* 60 (1945), 1401.

- Derryberry, M., 'Health is Everybody's Business,' *Public Health Reports*, 64 (1949), 1293.
- Foucault, M., *The Birth of the Clinic: an Archaeology of Medical Perception* (London: Tavistock, 1973).
- Hochbaum, G. M., 'Why People Seek Diagnostic X-rays,' *Public Health Reports*, 71 (1956), 377.
- Last, J. M., 'The Clinical Iceberg,' *Lancet*, 2 (1963), 28.
- Mechanic, D. and Volkart, E. H., 'Illness Behaviour and Medical Diagnoses,' *Journal of Health and Human Behaviour*, 1 (1960), 86.
- Parsons, T., *The Social System* (New York: Free Press, 1951).
- Peterson, J., *The Medical Profession in Mid-Victorian London* (Berkeley: University of California Press, 1978).
- Rosen, G., *The Specialization of Medicine: with Particular Reference to Ophthalmology* (New York: Froben, 1944).
- Rosenstock, I. M., 'Why People Use Health Services,' *Millbank Memorial Fund Quarterly*, 44 (1965), 94.
- Rosenstock, I. M. *et al.*, 'Why People Fail to Seek Poliomyelitis Vaccination,' *Public Health Reports*, 74 (1959), 98.
- Sand, R., *The Advance to Social Medicine* (London: Staples Press, 1952).
- Shapiro, A. K., 'A Contribution to a History of the Placebo Effect,' *Behavioural Science*, 5 (1960), 109.
- Smith, A., *The Wealth of Nations* (London: 1776).
- Stevens, R., *Medical Practice in Modern England: the Impact of Specialization and State Medicine* (New Haven: Yale University Press, 1966).
- Stevens, R., *American Medicine and the Public Interest* (New Haven: Yale University Press, 1971).

8

Medicine, Diet and Moral Regulation: Foucault's Impact on Medical Sociology

Bryan S. Turner

Introduction

Medical sociology occupies a peculiar location within sociology as a whole. It has enjoyed remarkable success particularly in North America as an applied field of sociology with special relevance to the training of medical practitioners and health workers generally. Medical sociology has also been highly successful in attracting government funds for research, again in the applied arena. The peculiarity, however, of medical sociology is that it has traditionally lacked any significant theoretical coherence and has contributed relatively little to the analytical and conceptual development of sociology as such. It had no significant foundation in classical sociology and unlike other sub-fields such as the sociology of religion, the classical founders of sociology had relatively little to contribute to the sociological analysis of health. One possible exception might be Emile Durkheim's study of suicide (Durkheim, 1951). Various attempts have been made to bring medical sociology more into the mainstream of the discipline of sociology by, for example, developing the sociology of health and illness, which was seen to have a much broader range than medical sociology, to be less overtly committed to the profession of medicine and more concerned with the philosophical underpinnings of the concepts of disease and illness. The creation of *Sociology of Health and Illness* in 1979 is one indication of such an attempt to broaden the theoretical relevance of medical sociology. The debate between either medical sociology or the sociology of health and illness not only concerned the intellectual standing of the sociological study of health issues but also raised a fundamental question about the relationship between sociology and medical science, and between medical practice and the role of sociological evidence and perspectives. This controversy reflected an earlier debate between sociology in medicine, which was seen to be dominated by medical values and practices, and the sociology of medicine, which was concerned with the nature of medicine as a professional activity and with the impact of medicine on society. Of course, this controversy is not specific to medical sociology because the social role of sociology is critical to the entire discipline but, given the social significance and power of the medical profession in Western societies, this debate has a particular urgency in medical sociology. The challenge to medical sociology is whether it can develop effective alternative causal or explanatory models which challenge the medical model as the dominant paradigm by which we understand and approach disease and sickness. By and large, sociologists have had a strong commitment to social medicine as an alternative to individualistic allopathic practice, and they have been significantly interested in alternative medical treatments as a critique of the assumptions of mainstream Western medicine (Salmon, 1984).

Perhaps the main exception to this claim that traditionally medical sociology lacked a significant analytical focus occurred in the work of Talcott Parsons, particularly in the analysis of the 'sick role' in his *The Social System* (1951). Parsons' approach to medical and health issues was attractive to sociology because it located sickness within a paradigm of deviance and social control. Given the importance of the sociology of deviance in the 1960s, many of Parsons' ideas about doctor/patient interaction, the nature of medical practice and the social character of sickness all found a ready audience in sociology. As we now know, Parsons' sick-role theory was eventually heavily criticized for its functionalist assumptions, its apparent commitment to the underlying values of the medical profession, its narrow focus on patient behaviour, its failure to address the notion of abnormal illness behaviour, and its cultural specificity (Holton and Turner, 1986). This critique of the sick-role as a useful sociological perspective on sickness was part of a general critical rejection of Parsonian sociology in the 1970s and 1980s. Although these criticisms have become part of the taken-for-granted culture of contemporary sociology, they should not obscure the fact that for a number of decades Parsons' approach to medical sociology provided a point of continuity and coherence within a discipline which is notorious for its fragmentation and internal controversy.

These introductory comments on the recent history of medical sociology now need to be qualified by two interesting developments. The first is the general impact of Michel Foucault's analysis of knowledge and power which has come to influence a wide variety of research topics and perspectives in the study of mental health and sickness since the publication in English of *Madness and Civilisation* (Foucault, 1967). The second crucial development, which is closely related to an interest in Foucault's social philosophy, is the tentative development of the sociology of the body as a theoretical underpinning for medical sociology. In this chapter I want to comment on these contemporary theoretical developments in sociology which I shall then illustrate by an examination of the development of nutritional theory and dietetics. The inter-disciplinary relationship between medical science and medical sociology within the context of a discussion of Foucault's approach to power and knowledge can then be considered.

Foucault and the Development of Medical Sociology

Foucault's reception within the English-speaking world was initially based upon his work on the history of psychiatry and the problem of madness in Western civilization. Because Foucault was clearly associated with the political interests of minority groups such as the mentally ill, prisoners and homosexuals, his contribution to sociology was seen to be a contribution to the study of social control. Shortly after the English publication of *Madness and Civilisation*, Thomas Szasz (1971) published *The Manufacture of Madness* and R. Boyers and U. R. Orrill (1972) edited the influential *Laing and Anti-Psychiatry*. R. D. Laing's influential *Sanity, Madness and the Family* had been published in 1964. In sociology the dominant paradigm of deviance and mental illness was so-called labelling theory which owed a great deal to the work of writers such as H. Becker in *Outsiders* (1963). In short, the context within which Foucault was launched within the English-speaking world was such that his original theories were received as a contribution to social control theory, within which the mentally ill were seen to be a socially deviant group who challenged the basic norms and values of society and who, as a consequence of being labelled deviant, were forced into careers of secondary deviance. Many of the concepts of the sociology of deviance, such as the notions of delinquent drift, deviancy amplification, criminal stereotypes and secondary deviance, were helpful in explaining delinquency (particularly among young males) and made a practical contribution to the understanding of the functioning of social work agencies; it was not until Foucault's later work on *Discipline and Punish* (1977) and the projected six-volume study of *The History of Sexuality*, which began in English translation in

1979, that a more subtle and comprehensive understanding of the real significance of Foucault began to emerge.

In retrospect it is now clear that Foucault made two major contributions to contemporary social science, namely an analysis of power and a contribution to the understanding of the emergence of the modern self through technologies. Foucault's analysis of power has proved particularly useful in understanding the functions of the medical profession, particularly the functioning of the clinic (Foucault, 1973). Foucault's theory of power was a critical reaction against both French Marxism and the existentialism of Sartre. Recent biographies of Foucault (Eribon, 1991) show that his preoccupation with his own homosexuality, his critique of Marxism and his involvement in the politics of the French academy did much to shape his theory of power. Foucault sought to challenge the Marxist conceptualization of power as a macro-structure such as the state which functioned to support capitalism and which was displayed through major public institutions such as the police, the law and state agencies. Such a view of power was central to the work of Louis Althusser who was the dominant Marxist theoretician of the state in the 1960s and the ideological state apparatus. By contrast, Foucault saw power as a relationship which was localized, dispersed and diffused through the social system, operating at a micro or covert level through sets of specific practices. Power is embodied in the day-to-day practices of the medical profession within the clinic, through the activities of social workers, through the day-to-day decision-making of legal officers, and through the religious practices of the church as they operate through everyday life in the confessional. This approach to politics had a particular message for radical Marxism, namely that the attempt to seize the state through political action would not destroy power, because power is rather like a colour dye diffused through the entire social structure and is embedded in daily practices. This view of power is very closely associated with Foucault's fascination for discipline, namely that power exists through the disciplinary practices which produce particular individuals, institutions and cultural arrangements. The disciplinary management of society results in a carceral, that is a form of society in which the principles of Bentham's panopticon are institutionalized in society through everyday arrangements. These ideas about power were further elaborated through Foucault's interest in 'governmentality', a system of power which articulated the triangular relationship between sovereignty, discipline and government. Governmentality (Foucault, 1991), which emerged in the eighteenth century, is a mechanism for regulating and controlling populations through an apparatus of security. This governmental apparatus required a whole series of specific *savoirs* and was the foundation for the rise of the administrative state (Gutting, 1989).

A further important feature of Foucault's work was the analysis of the relationship between power and knowledge. Whereas liberal theory tended to separate power and knowledge on the grounds that truth is always corrupted by the exercise of power, Foucault saw that power and knowledge were always inevitably and inextricably interconnected so that any extension of power involved an increase in knowledge and every elaboration of knowledge involved an increase in power. Foucault approached this question typically through a consideration of populations and bodies. For example, the growth of penology and criminology was closely associated with the development of panoptic principles of surveillance and control. In a similar fashion, the whole development of psychology and psychiatry was seen in terms of forms of knowledge, related to an extension of power over the subordinate populations of urban Europe. Foucault's very influential study of *The Order of Things* (1970) showed the intimate relationships between forms of surveillance and control and the development of social scientific knowledge. In fact Foucault normally spoke about knowledge in the plural (*savoirs*) in order to illustrate the notion that specific forms of power required highly specific and detailed formations of knowledge.

This conceptual apparatus which Foucault built up around the study of the history of ideas, the analysis of power, and the explication of forms of discipline proved enormously useful and important for medical sociologists in their attempt to understand the forms of power assumed by medical practices. Foucault's work permitted sociologists to think about the medicalization of society within a new framework, where the exercise of medical power was seen in terms of local diffuse practices. The influence of Foucault is particularly significant in such publications as *Political Anatomy of the Body: Medical Knowledge in Britain in the Twentieth Century* (Armstrong, 1983) and *Medical Power and Social Knowledge* (Turner, 1987a). The medical sociology which was inspired by Foucault is typically understood to be a distinctive break with the past. It was heavily informed by theoretical and philosophical analysis; it was highly critical of established medicine, seeking to provide alternative ways of examining mental illness and disease; it placed power and knowledge at the centre of the sociological understanding of medical institutions; and it showed how medical ideas of the moral character of disease operated at an everyday level. As Foucault's work evolved and as more of his studies were translated into English, such as *The Use of Pleasure* (1988a) and *The Care of the Self* (1988b), it also became clear that for Foucault the study of medicine was part of a larger programme which examined the evolution of sexuality in European societies from classical Greece onwards, and how that evolution was intimately bound up with the transformation of medicine. In his final publications Foucault appeared to turn more and more to an analysis of the self in the context of medical history and the development of sexuality. His interest in how the self in Western societies was an effect of discourse of the self became increasingly obvious in his studies of 'technologies of the self' (Martin *et al.*, 1988). Medical sociology and the sociology of health and illness were now seen to be both far broader in their terms of reference and also more central to the mainstream concerns of sociology as a whole. Specifically Foucault's particular approach to the sociology of knowledge was perceived as a distinctive departure from the legacy of Talcott Parsons.

Although Foucault's work is of enormous significance, it is not clear that the development of Foucaultian medical sociology was necessarily a total rupture with the past. I have argued on a number of occasions (Turner, 1987a; Robertson and Turner, 1991) that there is an important analytic relationship between Parsons' view of power as a medium of exchange and Foucault's approach to power as a set of micro-practices. Parsons also saw power as a diffused feature of all social systems and, like Foucault, thought that power was productive rather than negative. It is possible to argue from a sociological perspective that both Parsons and Foucault were providing a description of what one might call 'the institutions of normative coercion', such as the law, religion and medicine (Turner, 1992). These institutions are coercive in the sense that they discipline individuals and exercise forms of surveillance over everyday life in such a way that actions are both produced and constrained by them. However, such institutions as the medical clinic are not coercive in the violent or authoritarian sense because they are readily accepted as legitimate and normative at the everyday level. These institutions of normative coercion exercise a moral authority over the individual by explaining individual difficulties and providing solutions for them. In this sense we could say that medicine and religion exercise an hegemonic authority because their coercive character is often disguised and masked by their normative involvement in the troubles and problems of individuals. They are coercive, normative and also voluntary. When as an individual I am confronted by problems, I might typically approach a priest, a doctor or a social worker for help in resolving my difficulties. I enter into a quasi-contractual relation with such people in order to bring about a solution, but the solution has moral significance for my current and future behaviour. We can see how the concept of the sick role fits so well into such a framework. A sick role is a voluntary relationship with a doctor of a contractual character such that the patient accepts the authority of the doctor to bring about a desirable future state of health which involves the surrender of certain forms of freedom. Giving up smoking, reducing one's alcohol intake, eating less fat, and taking up jogging might be a typical recommendation for a suspected heart problem. This adoption of a sick role therefore involves moral obligations to change one's behaviour. In this sense there seems to be a certain continuity between Parsons' view of medicine as the production of patient submission and Foucault's view of the relationship between knowledge and power.

It can also be argued (Turner, 1984 and 1987b) that there was a certain continuity between Max Weber's study of rationalization as an historical process and Foucault's study of the emergence of discipline and punishment through a system of panoptic surveillance. In Weber's famous studies of the Protestant ethic (1930), we know that he saw the origins of much of contemporary rationalization in the religious practices of the early Protestant sects where discipline was combined with an anti-magical world-view. For Weber, the monastery and the army were the two great historical origins of modern rational discipline. There seems to be a similar view in Foucault who also made an important study of the role of military discipline in the whole evolution of Western rational practices. For Weber and Foucault, the body was the crucial target in the evolution of these regulative practices.

For Weber the rationalization of the body was brought about by the secular impact of Protestant forms of discipline, whereas for Foucault the normalization of the body was the outcome of new forms of knowledge and surveillance associated with the control of captive populations such as armies, prisoners and the mentally ill. The fact that Weber and Foucault should converge on a disciplinary theory of society through an analysis of the body is in one sense hardly surprising since both men were deeply influenced by the legacy of Nietzsche's critical philosophy. Recent studies of Weber have put an important emphasis on his dependence upon Nietzsche for an analysis of personality and life orders (Hennis, 1988). Foucault's dependence upon Nietzsche's theory of the will to power is obvious in the former's work on discipline, knowledge and power (Lemert and Gillan, 1982).

In an article in *Liberation* on 30 June 1984 Foucault had observed that 'we are all ruled, and as such, we are in solidarity' (Eribon, 1991: 279). This is an epigrammatic expression of his personal philosophy within which the problems of discipline and transgression were significant polarities which contained a strong Nietzschean legacy. The critique of modern medicine was that it represented a form of government which controlled individual transgression through a network of local normative constraints. It was an effective, localized institution of normative coercion to produce compliant patients.

Although there was significant evolution and change in Foucault's social philosophy, it is clear that the body and populations played a major role in the analytic structure of his work. The body was the focus of military disciplinary practices but it was also subject to the monastic regulation of medieval Catholicism. The body is also the target of the medical gaze and of governmentality generally. Health is a form of policing which is specifically concerned with the quality of the labour force. This view was very clearly expressed by Foucault in an article on 'The Politics of Health in the Eighteenth Century' where he suggested that it arguably concerns the economico-political effects of the accumulation of men. The great eighteenth-century demographic upswing in Western Europe, the necessity for co-ordinating and integrating it into the apparatus of production and the urgency of controlling 'it with finer and more adequate power mechanisms caused "population," with its numerical variables of space and chronology, longevity and health, to emerge not only as a problem but as an object of surveillance, analysis intervention, modification etc.' (Foucault, 1980b: 171) The nexus of knowledge/power was thus initially an effect of demographic changes, particularly the pressure of populations on systems of government and regulation from the eighteenth century. The body was clearly of major significance in *Discipline and Punishment*, but it also continued to play a crucial role in the larger project of *The History of Sexuality*, where Foucault was concerned with the body in relation to medicine and the body in relation to the development of the self within a Christian paradigm. Briefly Foucault was interested in the production of bodies, the regulation of bodies and the representation of bodies within a context of disciplinary surveillance. The integration of legal and medical controls over the body and identity was a theme in the study of hermaphrodites in *Herculine Barbin* (Foucault, 1980a). Foucault's work on the production of sexual identity played a major role subsequently in the historical analysis of gender and sexuality (Laqueur, 1990) and in the relationship between women and medicine (Martin, 1987). In subsequent years the sociology of the body emerged as a major theme in medical sociology because it provided a powerful perspective on the socially constructed nature of disease categories, the role of medicine in regulating individuals through regulating their bodies, and contributed also to new perspectives on the question of sexuality and medicine.

Having been neglected as a theoretical topic for many decades, the question of the human body has recently become a critical issue in the social sciences. There have been a number of major publications in this area resulting virtually in a new sub-field of sociology (Featherstone *et al.*, 1991; Leder, 1990; O'Neill, 1989; Shilling, 1993; Synnott, 1993). The causes and nature of this interest in the cultural aspects of the human body are both divergent and complex. However, this new interest in the body is clearly related to the growing problems of human identity brought about by legal and social changes which in turn are a consequence of technical transformations in medicine, specifically in the area of human reproduction. There is also widespread anxiety about the nature of contemporary epidemics such as HIV and AIDS which have drawn specific attention to the complexities of sexuality in modern society. These medical changes are also related to various social movements in modern society which seek to change social attitudes towards the body, particularly the gay and feminist movements. These anxieties about the body are also part of a broader concern about the demographic revolution of the last century, the process of ageing and the ecological deterioration of the environment. Within the context of capitalism, the body has also emerged as a significant feature in consumption advertising and consumer culture (Falk, 1994). Cultural postmodernization has also underlined the idea that the human body is simply a fabric or social product which has no ontological fixity. These postmodern questions about the body have brought a number of writers to speculate about the interaction between information systems, computer technology and the body. The employment of cyborgs in military activity and industrial production has been linked to science-fiction paradigms in which the socially produced body can be illustrated by such figures as Robocop and the supermen of the Terminator series (Haraway, 1990).

Research interest in the body is clustered around a number of domains. First, there is a wide interest in the symbolic importance of the body and the use of the body in representation as a metaphor of social relations. These approaches to the metaphoricality of the body owe a great deal to the anthropological work of Mary Douglas in *Purity and Danger* (1966) and *Natural Symbols* (1970). The issue of the asymmetrical nature of the body has been important in anthropological research on handedness, particularly in Robert Hertz's study of *Death and the Right Hand* (1960). Whether or not handedness has a specific relation to morbidity and mortality has been much debated (Coren, 1992), but the symbolic significance of the sinister side of the body cannot be ignored. Secondly, there is an interest in the active role of the body in shaping social relations and social reciprocity. As a generalization much of the sociological and anthropological literature on the body is concerned with what is done to the body, but there is an equally important question about what the body does to society. This particular approach has been much influenced by the phenomenology of Merleau-Ponty (1962) but Arthur Frank has produced an intriguing insight into the nature of illness which develops this perspective in his *At the Will of the Body* (1991). One criticism of Foucault in this area is that since he fully rejected any phenomenological or existentialist approach to the experience of embodiment, he all too frequently treated the body as merely an object. We need to develop a sociology of the body which will avoid such forms of dualism between the body as an object and as a subject.

The third area of sociological development is concerned with the whole problem of gender identity and sexuality in human societies, where feminist thought has obviously done much to question the taken-for-granted biological reductionism of earlier social theory. Foucault's work on the socially constructed nature of gender has been particularly important, and much work has been done on the impact of Christianity to the repression of sexual difference (Brown, 1988). This approach to the question of gender has been particularly important for medical sociology where the debate about anorexia nervosa has become a major topic for the development of an adequate sociology of the body (Brumberg, 1988). Alongside feminist theories of the body there has been an important development of gay theory in which the issue of masculinity has been brought into question with the same rigour which in previous generations was brought to bear on the question of femininity.

These and other developments have brought the question of the body to the forefront of much research in medical sociology. For example, the problem of the body in relation to medical categories lies at the base of the debate about social constructionism. Despite a number of promising developments in this area, many of the philosophical problems still remain unresolved, including the very basic question 'what is the body?' In order for the sociology of the body to flourish fully in the context of medical sociology we need a more coherent account of the basic ideas of the body, the objective body, embodiment and the history of the body. Although the sociology of the body is in many respects underdeveloped, it is clear that this approach to embodiment has a great potential for the analysis of pain, ageing, gender disorders, and disability (Scambler, 1987). The value of an embodied sociology is already obvious in the approach to death and ageing (Shilling, 1993) and to the study of pain (Scarry, 1985).

The Government of the Body: Social Policy and Obesity

Many of these theoretical and research developments in medical sociology can be illustrated by turning to some recent debates in social policy, concerning attitudes towards cholesterol and heart disease. The issue of diet and the body provides a useful focus for considering some implications of Foucault's work for the development of medical sociology and for social policy approaches to the human body in societies characterized by economic abundance.

I have suggested in the introduction to this chapter that medical sociologists, while often working alongside medics within a clinical setting, wanted to see themselves as critical observers of medical practice in institutions from the outside, as it were. This attempt to preserve a critical distance from medical practice was conducted under the guise of a commentary on sociology of medicine versus a sociology in medicine. In some respects it was Foucault who presented an interesting criticism of this alleged distance by suggesting that the earliest forms of social medicine were in fact sociological forms of research. For example, nineteenth-century enquiries into the health status of the working class which were undertaken by medical scientists were characteristically forms of sociological analysis on the impact of poverty, poor housing and harsh working conditions on the health status of the population. By taking this approach to social medicine, Foucault was able to demonstrate that the evolution of sociology was initially within the context of medical enquiry itself. Social medicine was a form of applied sociology, and hence the alleged distance between medicine and sociology was, at the very best, a twentieth-century disciplinary construction to show the autonomy of sociology within the academy. In *Medical Power and Social Knowledge* (1987a) I attempted to show that good medical practice would be necessarily sociological in attempting to locate individuals and groups within social space, and in a parallel fashion good investigative sociological enquiry into the health status of individuals would be something similar to a clinical enquiry into problems and difficulties of individuals. The disciplinary divisions between forms of academic enquiry are in this perspective an artifice of the university structure itself. I intend to illustrate this complicated relationship between social medicine, sociology and health policy through a brief overview of some aspects of the history of nutrition and diet (Crotty, 1994).

Medical practice, regardless of any claims about its scientific foundation in fundamental natural sciences, inevitably implies and embraces a moral view of both individuals and society, and therefore also engages in sociological reasoning. This combination of moral and social analysis can be neatly illustrated via a consideration of the etymology of the word 'diet.' As Foucault noted in *The History of Sexuality*, in classical Greek medical practice diet (*diata*) referred to a mode of living, that is, to the general conduct, structure and organization of individual life including an analysis of food, housing, dress and social relations. A diet prescribed a complete series of attitudes, beliefs, behaviour and conduct. Thus in classical Greek culture, the idea of a diet did not signify a limited or restricted set of eating practices, but rather embraced a general outline of life, society and politics. Diet was a critical feature of the Greek medical regime, where this regime was an ensemble of rules or practices imposed upon a person to achieve a status of well-being. Regime or regimen also has an antiquated meaning of government, and the term is the root of both regime and regiment. For example, a political diet in the Holy Roman Empire was a legislative assembly for the purpose of government. The *diata* was a general mode of living set within a government of the body which was to be achieved by prescribed medical practices. A well-disciplined or governed body, that is, a regulated body, within the context of a medical regime signifies the presence of discipline, moral organization, asceticism and self-control; by implication then the obese body signifies the absence of government and self-discipline. The unregulated body is a moral challenge to medical government. The obese and unregulated body represents a challenge to the social fabric of societies where personal asceticism is associated with moral stamina. This Greek medical perception of the body continued to influence Western medical practice and philosophy by its association with Christian theology, and hence in the work of medical writers like George Cheyne in the eighteenth century one finds this inter-weaving of medical and moral notions. It is hardly surprising that John Wesley, the Methodist leader, found Cheyne's views on diet an acceptable view of Christian personal behaviour (Turner, 1992).

If these nutritional views continued to have an impact on moral and medical belief, then it is interesting to note in addition that nutritional theories also found their way into Marxist philosophy via the work of Ludwig Feuerbach, who was important in the development of a materialistic perspective on human beings and society. Feuerbach had been influenced by nutritional theories which made popular the notion that 'man is what he eats.' The Feuerbachian view of human beings sought to criticize the idea of men as merely cognitive beings and attempted to promote a view of human beings as creative, sensuous, active agents involved in a dynamic relationship with their own external and internal environment. In this view, human beings are the outcome of their own productive activity in that they create themselves through labouring on their conditions of existence which include the activities of reproduction and consumption. This view of sensual human activity contributed in an important way to the development of Marxist materialism, in which men have to labour in order to live. Marxist humanism was in many respects grounded in a nutritional-moral view of human beings within which the material activity of production and reproduction had a critical focus. This Marxist reception of nutritional theory was a consequence of important scientific changes in theories of nutrition in the nineteenth century. By 1840, German chemists had successfully identified three chemical constituents of food, namely fats, proteins and carbohydrates, and they had begun to calculate with some precision the human requirements for each of these components. By the 1880s the scientific laws regarding the conservation of energy were then applied to living organisms, and scientists began to measure the potential energy in food and the energy which is expended by human labour in terms of calories, the unit which is used in thermodynamics to measure mechanical work. It was typical in the late nineteenth century therefore for scientists to regard food as a fuel for driving the human engine. It was this nutritional science that was applied to captive populations such as prisoners and the armed forces to measure the input requirements of certain human groups in order to achieve the most effective output of labour. These developments in nutritional science took place within the context of an industrial society in which political and economic leaders were concerned to improve the effectiveness and efficiency of labour by applying science to the domestic sphere. The aim of such campaigns was to reduce the cost of labour to capital by improving the efficiency of the working-class diet. These scientific campaigns therefore assumed a strong moral component in criticizing the 'irrationalities' of working-class diet.

One important illustration of such nutritional reform is the career of Wilbur Olin Atwater in the late nineteenth and early twentieth centuries. Atwater was one of the earliest dietary reformers to appeal to laboratory science for the legitimation of his social policy. Atwater's reformist career illustrates many of Foucault's arguments about the origins of social medicine in industrial policy. Atwater was a chemist who was well known for his laboratory nutrition in which he attempted to analyse foods to determine their composition, but he also undertook household food consumption surveys and measures of energy expenditure. He made numerous recommendations about the protein and energy requirements of human beings and developed tables of food composition, but he also applied these ideas to social problems. Atwater's works were also supported by Ellen Swallow Richards, who was a founder of the home economics movement in the United States. Atwater's reformist views of working-class diet were supported by his employer, the Wesleyan University in Middletown, Connecticut. His nutritional views were applied to industrial workers in Connecticut who were encouraged to buy cheap cuts of meat and inexpensive carbohydrate-rich diets alongside an encouragement to eat vegetables and fruits. One implication of Atwater's dietary regime was that the enjoyment of food was a privilege of the dominant classes while the workers were expected to be ascetic. Nutrition was thus seen to be an important aspect of scientific management since Atwater's dietary survey suggested that existing weight levels were sufficient to achieve a minimum protein and calorie requirement for workers if they learned to eat scientifically.

In the twentieth century nutrition continues to be closely associated with the achievement of national goals and with the creation of a healthy and happy population. During the First and Second World Wars, nutritional theories were significant in the development of domestic policy when eating appropriate food was seen by political leaders as an essential feature of the battle on the home front. However, these classical nutritional views were all developed in societies based upon some notion of scarcity. The importance of dietary regimes in the late twentieth century is that they have been formulated in societies based upon an assumption of abundance. Our dietary theories, especially concerning cholesterol levels, are couched in terms of an anxiety about obesity in a context of economic wealth and social abundance. In the post-war period men are dying, not from acts of violence in warfare, but from chronic disease brought about by obesity and a sedentary existence. This change in concern from under- to over-consumption of food can be dated from the United States Committee on the National Nutritional Plan of 1974. Americans were seen to be eating themselves to death because they lacked appropriate nutritional education. In the United States the McGovern Committee report was successful in connecting nutritional research with individual lifestyle needs of the middle classes who were the target of the nutritional reforms of the late twentieth century. These nutritional regimes not only recommended a reduction of saturated fat but also encouraged Americans to undertake regular exercise to offset the consequences of sedentary work. These nutritional theories of over-consumption and the policy of achieving a fat-reduced diet became interlinked with an ascetic view of thinness and female beauty.

In contemporary society the slogan 'eat less fat' works exceptionally well because it trades upon existing anxieties about the self and the body which are common in modern society, particularly for women. The representational self or the 'looking-glass self' is constituted by the reflection of the self in others. The appraisal of the self is now focused on the exterior image of the body in society. Being good is therefore closely associated with looking good, and looking good is defined by slimness and a regulated lifestyle producing an ascetic self-image. Body asceticism is designed to make an acceptable social self, particularly a self that gives off significant sexual symbolism. Looking good means looking sexually attractive, and for women this has become the dominant body image based upon the glamour of thinness. The modern psyche is expressed through the image of the body, that is, through a sexually charged body image. While the medical slogan 'eat less fat' may have been generated by nutritional research with the intention of proving the mortality and morbidity rates of advanced industrial societies, 'eating less fat' is socially acceptable in a popular culture because it is understood within a discourse of sexuality. The whole issue of diet is inextricably bound up with the problem of the modern personality. The negative side of this representational self is the evolution of anorexia nervosa as a predominantly female eating disorder which reveals and captures many of the underlying contradictions of contemporary culture.

The slimming industry and the fashion industry, which have embraced the image of the anorexic female as a norm of female beauty, have been the target of considerable feminist and sociological criticism. Suzie Orbach's *Fat is a Feminist Issue* (1978) gave rise to a significant literature on the political problem of diet in relation to the status of women in society. The subtitle of her book, the *Anti-Diet Guide to Permanent Weight Loss*, rather perfectly illustrates the critical tone of much feminist sociology in this field. Specific criticism of the impact of nutritional theories on class relations has also been developed by writers like Naomi Aronson (1982). The damaging implication of expert advice for women in the medical field has also been addressed by sociological theorists such as Ehrenreich and English (1978). Despite this critical response to nutritional theory and practice by sociologists, it is nevertheless the case, following Foucault's argument, that nutrition is a form of applied sociology and that the work of reformists like Atwater belongs to a tradition of social medicine and applied sociology. Given the relativistic implications of Foucault's argument, it is inevitable that any extension of power involves an extension of knowledge and that nutritional theory in relation to social classes is a particularly good illustration of this Foucaultian paradigm.

Conclusion: Theory and Practice

In a context of cultural postmodernism, much has been written recently about the idea of *post-histoire*, that is, the sense that history as a meaningful sequence of events has come to a conclusion. For many writers such as Jean Baudrillard there is a definite sense of the end of the social (Rojek and Turner, 1993). If sociology was that discipline which provided industrial modernity with a critical theory, then the disappearance or decline of industrialization as a principle of social organization must imply the disappearance of sociology. Certainly sociology is that discipline which provided us with the principal concepts and terminology for the analysis of industrial capitalism. Such concepts as the division of labour, social classes, rationalization and bureaucracy have fuelled the debate about Fordist industrialism. If modern forms of technology, communication and social arrangements have invented or created a new type of social order, then the classical terminology of sociology certainly looks dated, if not obsolete.

If such a perspective has any merit (and I think it does) then from a Foucaultian perspective, sociology was part of the whole apparatus by which industrial capitalism was to be managed, surveyed and regulated. It was part of the ensemble of disciplines by which governmentality was to be installed. Sociology was part of a network of disciplines which included criminology, penology, administrative sciences, and indeed social medicine, by which an industrial civilization was to understand itself and control subordinate social groups and classes. Although sociology's self-perception as a radical or critical discipline has been accepted by many, sociology is nevertheless part of the *savoirs* (to use Foucault's plural noun) for administrative knowledge by which industrial capitalism was to be understood and appropriated. Regardless of the critical and radical attitudes of many sociologists who entered the discipline in the 1960s and 1970s, sociology inevitably produces information about society which becomes part of the governmentality of the system as a whole. Furthermore, in this chapter, following Foucault's views on social medicine, sociology itself appears to be the product of the social reformist period of the nineteenth century, and nutritionists like Atwater contributed to the growth of a sociological approach to nutrition and social class which is a perfectly respectable part of the legacy of traditional applied sociology. Although sociology has played a valuable role in the critique of the medical model and provided a genuine social perspective on the nature of sickness, sociology is inextricably part of the academy which also houses medical science and related disciplines. Sociology is not in essence different from social epidemiology or social demography or social medicine. Of course, the claim which sociologists want to make is that their perception of the social world is in some sense more accurate, more detailed and more valid than other forms of knowledge. Were medicine to embrace fully a sociological perspective, the implication must be that we would have a better medical practice and superior medical institutions, more attuned to the needs of individuals and social groups. However, the implication of this argument is that medical power would be actually enhanced by the acquisition of a sociological perspective. The so-called problem of patient compliance would be a good example of this paradox. The argument of sociologists is that the lack of patient compliance is a consequence of poor medical understanding of the everyday world of the patient. Medical instructions and regimes are in some sense alien to this everyday world. The role of sociology in this argument would be to produce a better fit between medical ideas and everyday practice, but the consequence of such a better fit would of course be enhanced patient control by medicine. We could regard this as yet another version of the Foucault paradox (Abercrombie *et al.*, 1986: 189). The more individuals are individuated, separated and distinguished by the social process of individualism, the more they can be regulated, surveyed and controlled. Sociology is part of the more general process of rationalization by which advanced capitalism became administered in the nineteenth and twentieth centuries. Sociology was itself part of that government of the body which has characterized the history of western Europe through the application of medical principles to life as a whole.

References

- Abercrombie, N., Hill, S. and Turner, B. S. (eds), *Sovereign Individuals of Capitalism* (London: Allen and Unwin, 1986).
- Armstrong, D., *Political Anatomy of the Body: Medical Knowledge in Britain in the Twentieth Century* (Cambridge: Cambridge University Press, 1983).
- Aronson, N., 'Nutrition as a Social Problem. A Case Study of Entrepreneurial Strategy and Science,' *Social Problems,* 29 (5) (1982), 474–87.
- Becker, H. S., *Outsiders. Studies in the Sociology of Deviance* (Glen Coe: Free Press, 1963).
- Boyers, R., and Orrill, U. R.. *Laing and Anti-Psychiatry* (Harmondsworth: Penguin Books, 1972).
- Brown, P., *The Body and Society. Men, Women and Sexual Renunciation in Early Christianity* (London: Faber and Faber, 1988).
- Brumberg, J. J., *Fasting Goals. The Emergence of Anorexia as a Modern Disease* (Cambridge, Mass.: Harvard University Press, 1988).
- Coren, S., *Left-hander. Everything You Need to Know about Left-Handedness* (London: John Murray, 1992).
- Crotty, P., *The Good Nutrition. Culture or Science?* (Sydney: Allen and Unwin, 1994).
- Douglas, M., *Purity and Danger. An Analysis of Concepts of Pollution and Taboo* (Harmondsworth: Penguin Books, 1970).
- Douglas, M., *Natural Symbols. Explorations in Cosmology* (Harmondsworth: Penguin Books, 1973).
- Durkheim, E., *Suicide. A Study in Sociology* (Glen Coe: Free Press, 1951).
- Ehrenreich, B. and English, D., *For Her Own Good. 150 Years of the Experts' Advice to Women* (London: Pluto Press, 1978).
- Eribon, D., *Michel Foucault* (London: Faber and Faber, 1991).
- Falk, P., *The Consuming Body* (London: Sage, 1994).
- Featherstone, M., Hepworth, M. and Turner, B. S. (eds), *The Body. Social Process and Cultural Theory* (London: Sage, 1991).
- Foucault, M., *Madness and Civilization. The History of Insanity in the Age of Reason* (London: Tavistock, 1967).
- Foucault, M., *The Order of Things* (London: Tavistock, 1970).
- Foucault, M., *The Birth of the Clinic. An Archaeology of Medical Perception* (London: Tavistock, 1973).
- Foucault, M., *Discipline and Punish. The Birth of the Prison* (London: Allen Lane, 1977).
- Foucault, M., *The History of Sexuality, Volume 1: An Introduction* (London: Allen Lane, 1979).

- Foucault, M., *Herculine Barbin. Being the Recently Discovered Memoirs of a Nineteenth Century French Hermaphrodite* (Brighton: The Harvester Press, 1980a).
- Foucault, M., 'The Politics of Health in the Eighteenth Century,' in C. Gordon (ed.), *Power/Knowledge. Selected Interviews and Other Writings – 1972–1977* (Brighton: The Harvester Press, 1980b), 166–82.
- Foucault, M., *The History of Sexuality, Volume 2: The Use of Pleasure* (London: Allen Lane, 1988a).
- Foucault, M., *The History of Sexuality, Volume 3: The Care of the Self* (London: Allen Lane, 1988b).
- Foucault, M., 'Governmentality,' in G. Burchel, C. Gordon and P. Miller (eds), *The Foucault Effect* (Brighton: Harvester Wheatsheaf, 1991), 87–194.
- Frank, A., *At the Will of the Body. Reflections on Illness* (Boston: Houghton-Mifflin, 1991).
- Gutting, G., *Michel Foucault's Archaeology of Scientific Reason* (Cambridge: Cambridge University Press, 1989).
- Hennis, W., *Max Weber: Essays in Reconstruction* (London: Allen and Unwin, 1988).
- Hertz, R., *Death and the Right Hand* (London: Cohen and West, 1960).
- Holton, R. J. and Turner, B. S., *Talcott Parsons on Economy and Society* (London and New York: Routledge and Kegan Paul, 1986).
- Laing, R. D., *Sanity, Madness and the Family, Volume 1: Families of Schizophrenics* (London: Tavistock, 1964).
- Laqueur, T., *Making Sex. Body and Gender from the Greeks to Freud* (Cambridge, Mass.: Harvard University Press, 1990).
- Leder, D., *The Absent Body* (Chicago and London: Chicago University Press, 1990).
- Lemert, C. C. and Gillan, G., *Michel Foucault. Social theory and Transgression* (New York: Columbia University Press, 1982).
- Martin, E., *The Woman in the Body. A Cultural Analysis of Reproduction* (Milton Keynes: Open University Press, 1987).
- Martin, L. H., Guttman, H. and Hutton, P. H. (eds), *Technologies of the Self. A Seminar with Michel Foucault* (London: Tavistock, 1988).
- Merleau-Ponty, M., *Phenomenology of Perception* (London: Routledge and Kegan Paul, 1962).
- O'Neill, J., *The Communicative Body. Studies in Communicative Philosophy, Politics and Sociology* (Evanston: North Western University Press, 1989).
- Orbach, S., *Fat is a Feminist Issue. A Self-Help Guide for Compulsive Eaters* (New York: Paddington Press, 1978).
- Parsons, T., *The Social System* (London: Routledge, 1951).

- Robertson, R. and Turner, B. S. (eds), *Talcott Parsons. Theorist of modernity* (London: Sage, 1991).
- Rojek, C. and Turner, B. S. (eds), *Forget Baudrillard?* (London and New York: Routledge, 1993).
- Ryan, M. and Gordon, A., *Body Politics. Disease, Desire and the Family* (Boulder: Westview Press, 1994).
- Salmon, J. W., (ed.), *Alternative Medicines. Popular and Policy Perspectives* (London: Tavistock, 1984).
- Scambler, G., (ed.), *Sociological Theory and Medical Sociology* (London:Tavistock, 1987).
- Scarry, E., *The Body In Pain.The Making and Unmaking of the World* (New York: Oxford University Press, 1985).
- Shilling, C., *The Body and Social Theory* (London: Sage, 1993).
- Synnott, A., *The Body Social. Symbolism Self and Society* (London and New York: Routledge, 1993).
- Szasz, T. S., *The Manufacture of Madness. A Comparative Study of the Inquisition and the Mental Health Movement* (London: Routledge and Kegan Paul, 1971).
- Turner, B.S., *The Body and Society. Explorations in Social Theory* (Oxford: Blackwell, 1984).
- Turner, B. S., *Medical Power and Social Knowledge* (London: Sage, 1987a).
- Turner, B. S., 'The Rationalization of the Body. Reflections on Modernity and Discipline,' in S. Lash and S. Whimster (eds), *Max Weber, Rationality and Modernity* (London: Allen and Unwin, 1987b), 222–41.
- Turner, B.S., *Regulating Bodies. Essays in Medical Sociology* (London and New York: Routledge, 1992).
- Weber, M., *The Protestant Ethic and the Spirit of Capitalism* (London: George Allen and Unwin, 1930).

Index

HELENA EILSTEIN

Life Contemplative, Life Practical
An Essay on Fatalism

Amsterdam/Atlanta, GA 1997. 163 pp.
(Poznań Studies in the Philosophy of the Sciences and the Humanities 52)
ISBN: 90-420-0183-6 Bound Hfl. 70,-/US-$ 36.50

Contents: Acknowledgements. Preface. CHAPTER ONE: OLDCOMB AND NEWCOMB. 1. In the King Comb's Chamber of Game. 2. The Newcombian Predicaments. CHAPTER TWO: ANANKE. 1. Fatalism: What It Is Not? 2. Fatalism: What Is It? 3. Fatalism and *a priori* Arguments. 4. Fatalism and 'Internal' Experience. 5. Determinism, Indeterminism and Fatalism. 6. Transientism, Eternism and Fatalism. 7. Fatalism: What It Does Not Imply? CHAPTER THREE: FATED FREEDOM. 1. More on Libertarianism. 2. On the Deterministic Concept of Freedom. 3. Moral Self and Responsibility in the Light of Probabilism. 4. Fated Freedom. CHAPTER FOUR: THE VIRUS OF FATALISM. 1. Fatalism and Problems of Cognition. 2. The Virus of Fatalism: Why Mostly Harmless?

SEX, LOVE, AND FRIENDSHIP

Studies of the Society
for the Philosophy of Sex and Love, 1977-1992

Ed. by Alan Soble

Amsterdam/Atlanta, GA 1997. LII,644 pp.
(Value Inquiry Book Series 45)
ISBN: 90-420-0001-5 Bound Hfl. 350,-/US-$ 180.-
ISBN: 90-420-0227-1 Paper Hfl. 90,-/US-$ 47,-

This collection joins together sixty essays on the philosophy of love and sex. Each was presented at a meeting of The Society for the Philosophy of Sex and Love held between 1977 and 1992 and later revised for this edition. Topics addressed include ethical and political issues (AIDS, abortion, homosexual rights, and pornography), conceptual matters (the nature, essence, or definition of love, friendship, sexual desire, and perversion); the study of classical and historical figures (Plato, Aristotle, Spinoza, Kant, and Kierkegaard); and issues in feminist theory (sexual objectification, the social construction of female sexuality, reproductive and marital arrangements). Authors include Jerome Shaffer, Sandra Harding, Michael Ruse, Richard Mohr, Russell Vannoy, Claudia Card, M.C. Dillon, Gene Fendt, Steven Emmanuel, T.F. Morris, Timo Airaksinen, and Sylvia Walsh. The editor, who is the author of Pornography (1986), The Structure of Love (1990), and Sexual Investigations (1996), has also contributed six pieces and an Introduction.